Praise for Sex A̶

"Joan Price has crossed taboo boundaries again—this time about the impact on sex of loss and grieving. All of us who cope with rebirthing sex after facing loss of a beloved wish we had a roadmap to follow. This book lights a path that sets us on the journey to recovery, with content that is relevant, necessary and inspiring for grievers and the helping professionals that serve them. It is truly a gift to humankind!"

—Patti Britton, PhD, co-founder of SexCoachU.com, known worldwide as the *Mother of Sex Coaching*

"Price's latest book begins a much-needed conversation on what has long been considered a taboo question: what happens to your sex life after the death of a partner? Price offers valuable advice and guidance in an accessible writing style that brims with passion and compassion."

—Dr. Justin Lehmiller, author of *Tell Me What You Want: The Science of Sexual Desire and How It Can Help You Improve Your Sex Life*

"Joan Price is one of the smartest thinkers around about sex, regardless of your age—or hers!"

—Dan Savage

"With her characteristic clarity and insight, senior sexpert Joan Price zeros in on an experience that many people navigate but very few discuss: the experience of reclaiming sex after the death of a beloved. *Sex After Grief* is a profoundly compassionate, deeply personal, and exceptionally practical guidebook for moving forward after loss with both purpose and joy."

—Lynn Comella, PhD and author of *Vibrator Nation: How Feminist Sex-Toy Stores Changed the Business of Pleasure*

"Deeply, honestly sourced in her own experience but aware that other people's mileage may vary, this wise, compassionate, moving, sex-positive, and so necessary book breaks silence and lucidly tackles an all-too-common source of pain and shame. Author Joan Price has stitched 'patches of [her] grief quilt' together with other bereaved lovers' insights and experiences woven throughout.

It will prove a source of comfort for those who are grieving, and advice and support for those who are ready to open back up to sex, pleasure and love."

—Carol Queen PhD, Good Vibrations sexologist, co-founder of Center for Sex & Culture, San Francisco

"I always love Joan's books because they are real, honest, inspirational, and audacious. *Sex After Grief* will advise and surprise you, whatever your age, gender, or orientation."

—Betty Dodson, PhD, author, artist, sexologist, orgasm educator since the early 1970s

Sex After Grief

Sex After Grief: Navigating Your Sexuality After Losing Your Beloved

Library of Congress Cataloging-in-Publication number: 2019938544
ISBN: (p) 978-1-68481-602-6 (e) 978-1-68481-603-3
BISAC category code: FAM014000, FAMILY & RELATIONSHIPS / Death, Grief, Bereavement

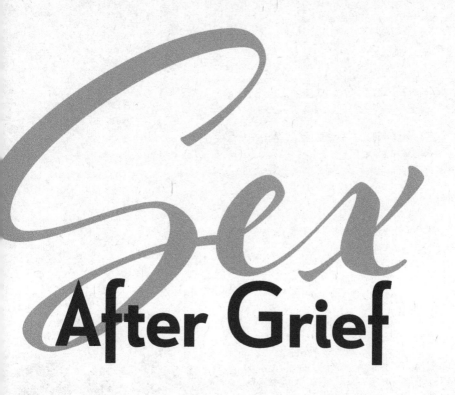

After Grief

Navigating Your Sexuality After
Losing Your Beloved

JOAN PRICE

Author of the award-winning
Naked at Our Age: Talking Out Loud about Senior Sex

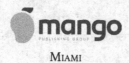

mango
PUBLISHING GROUP

MIAMI

I dedicate this book to:

- My great love, Robert Rice, who lives in my memory and in my heart.

- Mac Marshall, who shows me that joy is possible after grief.

- All the grievers who generously shared their stories and opened their hearts so that this book could happen.

Table of Contents

Introduction to the 2024 Edition

"I finished reading *Sex After Grief* in a day. What an absolute difference this book made for me! I had felt shame about my sexual thoughts and feelings so soon after my husband's passing. I was going crazy with the weight of my guilt, and, at the same time, lust was crushing me. Reading this book was like finding water in the desert. I feel less alone in my struggles."

—*Sex After Grief* reader

What follows in this book is the original *Sex After Grief* (chapters 1–17), plus four new chapters. *Sex After Grief* came out in 2019 to rave reviews, praise from readers, and many grateful emails from grievers. It won the 2020 Service/Self-Help Book Award from the prestigious American Society of Journalists and Authors. I regularly speak on this topic to groups of seniors, bereaved of all ages, therapists, podcasters, and news media internationally.

Why revisit the book in 2024 and add new content? The first edition spoke mainly to people who were in the process of starting to date again after their loss. Some had new loves already. Some were hoping. Many were anxious, reluctant, and confused by their sexual feelings. Five years later, how are those grievers now? Are their relationships still intact and fulfilling? What additional information do grievers need about how to navigate new relationships over time? From the many questions you ask me, I realized I needed to add more to this book on topics like these:

- Can we love another person and our deceased beloved at the same time? What does that look like?

- How do we make the best choices in partners and relationship styles for this stage of our lives?

- How do we keep sex satisfying after first lust has worn off?

- If love happens and we're riding the joy of life again, how do we cope when the wheels fall off?

- How do we continue to move forward, keeping our beloved still strong inside us, while opening ourselves up to new experiences and new partners?

Joan's Dream of Robert

I dreamed of Robert for the first time in years. He was an angel! He was flying, swooping in the sky, huge wings gracefully dancing. He didn't see me and was flying away. I called out, but he didn't hear me. So I—much less gracefully—started to fly, too! I wasn't very good at it, and the distance between us grew. I've got to catch him! I must hold him again! *These panicked thoughts propelled me to fly faster, and I caught up to him. He turned to me, smiled his tender lover's smile, eyes soft. He enfolded me in his arms and kissed me. Then he looked at me, staring his artist's stare, and slowly caressed my face. He was beautiful, the Robert of our first years together. He wrapped me in his arms again, so close that I couldn't tell which body was his and which was mine. He kissed me, a long kiss, the gentle kind he called a "sweet kiss." I woke with tears on my cheek.*

"What is it like for you returning to *Sex After Grief* and writing new chapters?" Rae Francoeur, a dear writer friend, asked me.

"It's wonderful—I love it," I told her. "When I was writing *Sex After Grief* in 2019, I cried through much of it."

"I remember," said Rae.

"But now, there's pure joy in sharing new stories and new perspectives. I think I've healed!" I paused. "The only part that made me cry this time was writing my dream of Robert."

I realize now that I cried more from the beauty of reconnecting with Robert than from the loss. I carry Robert in me when I dance, when I teach, when I learn, when I move in the world.

I wish the same for you. I hope this book helps you, wherever you are in your grief journey right now. Know that whatever you're feeling or wanting, you're not alone.

—Joan Price

CHAPTER 1

Why a Book about Sex and Grief?

"I started to search for confirmation that my feelings were not inappropriate. What I found instead was a culture of silence. I read Joan Didion's and Joyce Carol Oates's classic memoirs about mourning a beloved husband. They are lauded as unflinching, but in their combined nearly seven hundred pages, there is no mention of the type of sexual bereavement I was experiencing. The unspoken message, as I received it: Keep your mouths shut about sex. I turned to self-help books for widows, and found that there, too, discussions about sex were pretty much nonexistent."

—Alice Radosh, "Taboo Times," in *Modern Loss: Candid Conversation about Grief. Beginners Welcome* by Rebecca Soffer and Gabrielle Birkner

There are many books about grief after loss of a beloved, but they almost never talk about sex. As research for this book, I read or perused dozens of contemporary books specifically about grief after death of a spouse or beloved partner. Almost none of them mentioned sex, and of those that did, rarely more than a page was about this important part of life. It's time to talk out loud about sex and grieving.

My love affair with Robert Rice was the reason I decided to write about sex and aging at age sixty-one with *Better Than I Ever Expected: Straight Talk about Sex After Sixty*. Over fourteen years, one book turned into four—and this one makes five. Senior sex education in its many forms—books, articles, my blog (www.nakedatourage.com), speaking engagements, Q and A column, webinars, a newsletter—became my mission and my life.

But when my second book, *Naked at Our Age: Talking Out Loud about Senior Sex*, was just a glimmer in my eye and two pages of notes, Robert—by then my husband—died. Died. Died. Died. That word insists that I write it again and again, as if the word is animate and claws repeatedly at my heart and my tear ducts.

My grief journey has lasted more than ten years as I write this book at age seventy-five. I've gone from such intense wailing, sobbing, and keening that I couldn't leave the house to living with joy again, becoming capable of laughter and intimacy once more, and letting a new, dear person into my heart. During that time, I cycled through a roller coaster of despair before learning to be a fully alive, sexual being again.

Many people helped me in my grief journey. I pay it forward by helping others. Part of that debt repayment, I realize, needs to be a book with this narrow focus: *How do we become capable of sex and intimacy when the person we want most to share this with is dead?* How do we find our way to letting someone else in? How do we know when we're ready? Is there one way that works for everyone?

The easy answer to that last question: No. We all experience grief in our own way, and that includes the myriad ways that we invite sex into our lives, or don't, and we change along the way. We all respond differently, and, as you'll hear me say throughout this book, however you respond is normal.

Some people feel frenetic sexual energy and yearn for a sexual outlet right away. Some start dating immediately, some gradually, some not ever. Some withdraw from sexual possibility. Some share their bodies but not their hearts. Many give themselves sexual release to the fantasy of their lost loved one. You'll meet many of these people in this book, whom I've named "Grievers," as they open their private lives and thoughts to you. I hope you'll come away realizing that no one is wrong and no choice is defective or shameful. You'll learn many options, and you will choose for yourself.

You'll read about some options that are clearly not your style or don't fit your beliefs. Please avoid condemning others who choose those paths. There's a difference between saying, "This would not be right for me," and "You shouldn't do this either."

As a writer, I documented most of my own changes as I struggled in grief, sometimes as public writing, often as private journaling. Other grievers shared their stories with me and continue to do so, and I know you'll learn much from them. Grief counselors were essential to my journey. I took notes after my sessions, and I share some of their wise suggestions with you. Excerpts from all these patches of my grief quilt are in this book to inform and help you.

I could not have written or even envisioned this book ten years ago, five years ago, or even two years ago. It took experiencing my grief journey fully, trying in many diverse ways to integrate my sexuality with my loss, and finally reaching an equilibrium that became not only acceptable but joyful. At this point, I feel ready to share my intimate journey with you in hope that it will help you as you experience your own.

I'm known as a writer and speaker about older-age sexuality. This book is mostly, but not exclusively, from a senior perspective. If you're younger, 80 percent of it will speak to you and give you information you won't find elsewhere. If you're not grieving but are dating someone who has lost a partner, you'll understand that person better. If you're a therapist whose bereaved clients come to you with their sexual longings, guilt, or desires, I hope you'll put this book in their hands after reading it yourself.

If you're a griever, parts of this book may make you cry, whether your grief is fresh or well-seasoned. It did that to me, writing it. As a sex educator and a grief survivor who has acquired some wisdom along the way, I feel it's my mission to write this book. If it helps you, I hope you'll let me know. You can reach me at joan@joanprice.com.

Your Takeaway

What questions do you hope this book
will answer?

CHAPTER 2

Myths about Sex and Grieving

"Day after day, you must endure the misguided comments from well-meaning people who just don't have a clue...There are those who say just the right thing; others who are well-meaning but stumble because they don't know better; and others who say or do things that are deeply hurtful."

—Patrick O'Malley, PhD, in *Getting Grief Right: Finding Your Story of Love in The Sorrow of Loss*

You'll probably have to deal with people who judge or shame or worry about you because of your personal choices. You'll be judged by people who think you're dating too quickly or moving into sex with a new person too fast. You'll be judged for remaining celibate.

Advice from friends and family can be helpful, but not always. Even when well-intentioned, advice that clamps down your sexuality can stall your healing and make you feel ashamed of your feelings and your body's desires. Likewise, advice that pushes you forward before you're ready can make you feel like you're doing grief wrong.

It's better to get your advice from a sex-positive therapist, grief counselor, or hospice worker. By "sex positive," I mean that they see sex as a normal and healthy part of life. They support you when you're ready to open up to sex again, acknowledging that there's no time frame that is right for everyone. (See Chapter 16, **Grief Counselors, Sex Coaches, Support Groups** for more.)

"Friends try to comfort with words
But they are taking my experience
and writing their own on top
Like an artist painting oil over watercolor."

—Susan Jean LaMaire, in "Seven Stages Scrambled" in *Chicken Soup for the Soul: Grieving and Recovery*

Myths Others Tell Us

Here are examples of myths about sex and grief. Some you may hear from people in your life or read in magazine articles. Others are beliefs you may have internalized about how grief works. Realize that these are *myths*, not truths.

Myth: It's not really sex you're missing: it's touch. Hug a friend or get a massage.

Truth: Sure, you're missing touch. But you're also missing sex: touch + arousal + orgasm.

"These [self-help books for widows] urged me not to confuse missing touch (acceptable) with missing sex (misguided). Missing touch didn't have anything to do with sex, I was told, and could be replaced with massages, cuddling grandchildren, and even going to hair salons to get shampoos. Clearly, they didn't know what Bart was like in bed. This loss wasn't something a hairdresser could handle."

—Alice Radosh, "Taboo Times," in *Modern Loss: Candid Conversation about Grief. Beginners Welcome* by Rebecca Soffer and Gabrielle Birkner

Myth: Wait at least a year before having sex with a new partner.

Truth: Sex is comforting and an outlet for your powerful emotions and needs. There's nothing wrong with you if you want to have sex soon after your beloved's death, or even the day after the funeral. The one-year rule is useful for most decision making—such as marrying again or mixing finances—but when you have first sex with a new person is entirely up to you and your willing sex partner.

Myth: Sex with someone new is disloyal to your deceased loved one.

Truth: Guilt, especially survivor's guilt, is a powerful force, but letting it rule our actions only harms us. Maybe you took the vow to be faithful "until death do us part." You didn't promise "after death for eternity thereafter." It's a horrible fact that your mate is gone, and nothing you do to care for yourself is "disloyal." Wouldn't your mate want you to care for yourself?

A Griever Shares

"Many people disapprove of a recently bereaved spouse jumping into the dating/mating game quickly. I was told by more than one person that it was 'appropriate' to wait a year before having sex with anyone. I thought that was bullshit, especially because my dear wife repeatedly urged me, 'Don't become a hermit' and 'Embrace life fully.' It became a mantra that she uttered over and again to me in her final months."

Myth: Wait until you're sure this new person is a potential next mate before having sex.

Truth: This may be true for you if you have firm religious convictions that only allow sexual expression within marriage. Otherwise, screening a possible sex partner as a potential next spouse will only create impossible hurdles and anxiety and send potential dates running. (See Chapter 5, **Dating Again,** for a more realistic approach.)

Myth: You need to get out there and should have started dating by now.

Truth: When people push you to start dating before you're ready, it says more about them than about you: your grief is making them uncomfortable, or they don't understand grief at all. Don't let yourself be influenced by anyone else's notion of when you should be ready.

Myth: You should wait until you're no longer grieving.

Truth: There is no magic moment when grief is over. Grieving is not finite. It does get easier and less painful over time, and it changes into a feeling and a deep connection you can live with. But there's no magical end point. Grief can coexist with desire—even love—for a new person.

"The thing about grief is that there isn't a place or time at which we arrive once-and-for-all at peace, or healing, or completion."

—Joanne Cacciatore, PhD in *Bearing the Unbearable: Love, Loss, and the Heartbreaking Path of Grief*

A Polyamorous Perspective

A perspective from David Wraith, sex educator, cofounder of Sex Positive St. Louis

Almost all the support, advice, and conventional wisdom around grieving the loss of a spouse or romantic partner is tailored to monogamous people. My grief support group was invaluable to me after my wife died, but I had to take a lot of their advice with a polyamory-flavored grain of salt. I was the only nonmonogamous person in my group, and even though I was among the most recently widowed, I was the only person who had dated anyone since my spouse's passing. Some of the others in the group had been widowed for years and still weren't ready to date.

One piece of advice that was shared in the group was, "You'll know you're ready to date again when you take off your wedding ring." My current partner and I have been together for three years, and I still wear my wedding ring. I wore it when I was dating other people when my wife was alive, so why take it off now?

One advantage to being queer, black, kinky, and polyamorous is that I'm used to having to screen mainstream thought and opinion through my own personal filter before applying it to myself. Being a polyamorous widower is no different. I had to expect and brace myself for the judgment of my monogamous friends for "dating again so soon," since many of them had no idea I was dating other people when my wife was still alive.

How Do You Respond to People Who Challenge Your Choices?

If they're close friends, tell them the truth about your reasons—or don't. If they're casual friends, feel free not to respond, or, if you prefer, shut them down. If they're hurtful or toxic, shut them down and/or avoid conversations with them. Some examples of responses you might give:

- I grieved a long time while my partner was ill. It's time for me to live again.

- I'm not ready to date yet. I'll know when I am.

- I'm moving forward on my own timetable. This doesn't need fixing.

- I'm perfectly capable of making my own decisions.

- I know you're concerned about me, but you don't need to be.

- We have differing opinions about what I should do.

- I know that worked for you, but we're not the same.

- That's private, thank you for your concern.

- I'll let you know if I need your advice, thanks.

- That's not helpful.

"The process cannot be hurried by friends and family, who may want to 'fix' a widow or widower by arranging a new relationship for them. However well-meaning this is, it frequently ends in disaster, because recovery and adjustment can take much longer than most people realize. Equally, friends can be judgmental and critical if they believe a bereaved person has gotten over the death of their partner too quickly and is dating someone new before an 'acceptable' amount of time has passed."

—Julia Samuel, in *Grief Works: Stories of Life, Death, and Surviving*

Myths We Tell Ourselves

Sometimes the myths that hold us back are those we've internalized. We feel guilty because we've bought into beliefs that honestly don't serve us anymore, if they ever did. For example:

Myth: Casual sex or sex with multiple partners is wrong and shameful.

Truth: You are an adult, fully capable of making your own decisions about what sex means to you, how you want to conduct your sex life, and with whom. There are myriad options for expressing our sexuality, and we can give ourselves permission for choosing the way that works for us now. Nothing you desire is wrong as long as it is consensual, safe, and honest. Choose your partners wisely and use safe sex protection every time.

Myth: Masturbation is wrong.

Truth: Masturbation is a wise choice for experiencing sexual release and all the good things that come with it—easier sleep, better mood, a lower likelihood of jumping into the wrong relationship out of sexual frustration. It's a way to be sexual without involving anyone else. (See Chapter 4, **Solo Sex.**)

Myth: If I choose my next partner carefully, I don't have to worry about sexually transmitted infections (STIs).

Truth: Use barrier protection always, with everyone. Please view my free "Safer Sex for Seniors with Joan Price" webinar on YouTube.

Myth: Nobody would want to have sex with me anyway.

Truth: That's depression talking. You may see yourself as undesirable right now because you're suffering too much to engage with another person. That's valid—you're not ready. But if you think no one would want you because you're too old or not in shape, please question that age-shaming, body-shaming attitude. It will only hold you back.

Myth: We can only love once. I'm done now.

Truth: It may feel like you can only love once, but many of us have discovered that loving deeply and completely does not prevent us from loving again. It will feel different, but it will be equally real.

> "You will lose someone you can't live without, and your heart will be badly broken, and the bad news is that you never completely get over the loss of your beloved. But this is also the good news. They live forever in your broken heart that doesn't seal back up. And you come through. It's like having a broken leg that never heals perfectly—that still hurts when the weather gets cold, but you learn to dance with the limp."
>
> **—Anne Lamott**

Your Takeaway

Which myths have interfered with you moving forward in your own way? Create your own response to people who try to advise or judge you in an unwelcome way.

CHAPTER 3

My Own Struggle with Sex After Grief

"Yes, the first year is the hardest, except for, in their own way, all the others."

—Gabrielle Birkner in *Modern Loss: Candid Conversation about Grief. Beginners Welcome.*

I'm a sex educator, author, blogger, public speaker. You'd think that with all I know about sex and how much I value it, I would have had an easy transition back into sex myself after Robert died. Not so! Even though I wrote about sex during that time, it took me months to feel sexual stirrings and begin pleasuring myself, and years to become sexual with a partner. Yes, *years!*

The last time Robert and I made love was three months before he died in August 2008. From the time Robert became too ill for sex through the first three months after his death, I felt no sex drive whatsoever and no sexual connection to my body. I couldn't imagine wanting to have another man touch me, nor did I have any desire to touch myself. My collection of vibrators stayed in a drawer. My only sex fantasies were memories of Robert as a healthy, loving, and enthusiastic sex partner. These memories led to great, gulping tears, not arousal.

Five months after Robert's death, I had a dream, which I recorded in my journal:

> *Jan. 5, 2009: I was with a new man, a stranger. He was behind me, his arms around my waist, and suddenly I could feel his erection through our clothes. I felt the stirrings of a sexual tingle, then I woke up and discovered I really was aroused! I sat up in bed, calling out, "I'm alive!"*

I marveled at the time that my dormant sexuality was suddenly waking up. Amazingly, it would take three more years before I would welcome another human being into my body, and longer than that before I could do that joyfully. Along the way, I tried to date, have sex with a buddy, date, have sex with a former lover, date some more...but it was like a slow train that had its own schedule. Nothing I tried to do changed some mysterious, inner timetable.

Fritz (Not His Real Name)

Fritz, a handsome, smart, accomplished male friend, was my confidant and buddy during the worst of my grieving period, and our close connection remains. He had known Robert and felt protective and compassionate after Robert died. We engaged in a routine of frequent walks, dinners, and candid talks. We often talked about love and sex. I enjoyed his maleness and openness, and I found myself flirting with him one moment, and in the next breath telling him a memory of Robert, whom he greatly admired.

After months of this comforting, platonic friendship, and just a week after my "arousal dream," a goodnight kiss turned into a lingering kiss, and yowza! My sexual electricity turned on and started buzzing my brain!

We took it slowly over months, sometimes letting our kisses and hands explore, sometimes not. We got to an "almost" stage, and he pulled back. I said yes. He said no. He didn't want to risk sacrificing our close friendship if we became sexual together. I assured him that we would be even better friends with sex in the mix. After a few more truncated explorations, we stopped, despite my protestations that we could have both friendship and sex. He felt protective of my vulnerability and, I realize now, his own. We returned to being platonic friends who talked plenty about sex but didn't explore it together.

I asked Fritz if he would be willing to share his perspective. He wrote this, and I'm grateful to him for his willingness to share it with you:

In Fritz's Words

"Ah, yes, we could have, maybe should have,
captured the moment, but there was risk.
Though mere frivolity would be fine, we were

too closely aligned not to expect a deeper emotional bond. Joan felt ready to reengage with love and life, yet her tears of loss were still present. It was early on, and Robert's welcome shadow lingered over us.

"There was no question of our dear love and openness with one another. It was something to protect and cherish in its innocence and honesty. Would sex corrupt us? Was I a temporary reprieve? Replacement? Did this matter, as the immediacy of sexual gratification quickened? Would our sexual activity reengage Joan in life, moving her forward—or would she incur a destabilizing setback? Could I commit to the heightened responsibility for Joan's emotional well-being which would clearly come with our lovemaking? Was I merely an opportunist, predatory and depraved? Could I expect a reciprocal level of support and responsible behavior from Joan as I widened my heart to someone so recently challenged by serious—almost existential—loss?

"No right or wrong here, but there clearly was risk of disruption, drama, hurt, and regression."

Trying to Date

Thirteen months after Robert's death, I made it a goal to meet new men and start dating. I went to dances and singles events. I joined Meetup singles groups. I signed up with Match.com and OkCupid and scoured Craigslist personals ads.

My first attempts at meeting new people were furtive and sad. I cried on the way home from first dates. I kept alternating between attempts at meeting new men and retreating.

Then I made dating a project. I developed my successful workshop, "How the Heck Do I Date at This Age?" because we teach what we need to learn, and by now I had plenty of experiences and tips to share. I realized that dating can be fun, and even bad dates make good stories. (See Chapter 5, **Dating Again**.)

I had more success with online dating after deciding to date widowers only. This was valuable in helping me get out of my hard, protective shell, but I didn't have anything in common with the men I met other than being widowed. So I relaxed that requirement, and lots of coffee dates and walking dates with new people followed. Many were interesting, but I didn't meet anyone whom I wanted to see naked.

At the time, I worried that I was handling this getting-back-to-dating process all wrong. Now I realize it wasn't wrong. I couldn't know when I was ready without trying, retreating, and trying again. Not everyone does it this way—there are no wrong ways to do grief—but that was my pattern.

Sometimes Sex Happened

In early 2012, three and a half years after Robert's death, I was finally able to have full partnered sex with a friend from another city who had been an occasional lover before I met Robert. He was sexually attentive and generous, but I was able to have an orgasm with him only by fantasizing that it was Robert. (I've since learned that this is quite common.) Afterward, I tried to fight the tears. I don't remember if I was successful.

Later on, I met a man who made me giddy-excited. The distance between our cities and his consuming job made dating difficult, and we only had a few dates. The last was sexual in non-penetrative ways and very sweet. I was surprised when he faded out of reach, claiming that he was too busy and his job stretched him too far.

You'll learn more about my sex-after-grief journey in other chapters of this book. For example,

- A spectacular, erotic massage that awakened my sexuality in a safe, nonreciprocal way. (Chapter 13, **Massage or More?**)

- Anticipation of sex with another former lover from many years ago, but, when we were in bed together, I couldn't do it. (Chapter 7, **It's Okay If You're Not Ready.**)

- Three dates with a good man I enjoyed and opened up to. We had one marvelous sex date. (Chapter 9, **It's Not All or Nothing.**)

- Reconnection with a former lover who became my sex buddy for more than two years. (Chapter 11, **Friends with Benefits**.)

And When It Works...

In 2017, OkCupid brought me a man who had just lost his wife after a long illness. He needed to learn to live with joy again, and this included sex. Our first date was instant attraction, and we discovered that we had many qualities, interests, and core beliefs in common. He was brainy, fit, attractive, and physically and intellectually active. He thought my work was fascinating.

A flurry of emails followed our first date as we tried to learn all we could about each other. In one, he asked, "Can you imagine having sex with me?"

I replied, "I'm imagining it now."

We became sexual on our second date. Two years later, we're still enjoying each other. We call each other "date mates," which to us means that we're in a strong, sweet, bonded relationship but have no desire to marry or move in together.

What I Learned from My Halting Steps

- We may not know when we're ready for sex.

- We don't have to have it all figured out.

- We should accept our emotional timetable, whatever it is.

- There may *not* be a magic moment when we know we're ready for sex.

- Kissing a friend can be a great start to getting back in touch with our sexual selves, even if it doesn't lead anywhere. (I know that won't work for everyone!)

- If we try and it doesn't work, that's not failure—it's all progress.

- When it does work, it can be glorious.

Your Takeaway

What has your struggle been so far in trying to
bring sex back into your life? Make your list of
the steps you took, the people you got naked with,
and the people you decided not to. What can you
learn about what you want and need from the
steps you've taken?

CHAPTER 4

Solo Sex

Y ou don't need a partner to receive an orgasm.
If you've got fingers and/or a well-chosen sex
toy, you can do it for yourself.

I know, you may long for human contact, the
warmth of another body, the shiver of excitement
from the unpredictability of a person's touch,
the cuddling after sex. But we don't always have
control over whether we have a desirable and
willing partner to give us those sensations and
pleasures. The special challenges of grief are
that we may not feel ready for a partner, despite
desiring sex, or that we may not have an available
partner if we do feel ready.

The best insurance for later-life quality of sex is
to stay sexually active with our own hands and
sex toys, especially when we're unpartnered, even
when we're grieving.

A Griever Shares

"During the final three sexless years of my wife's life while I was her full-time caregiver, had it not been for solo sex, I'd have gone stark raving bonkers and would've been wrapped up in a straitjacket and stuck in an institution. Masturbation kept me going."

Orgasm Benefits

Did you know that sexual activity and orgasm—no partner required—help elevate your emotional and physical health? When we grieve, our stress is up, our mood is down, our sleep is disturbed, we're depressed, and our overall health is compromised. All of these problems and more are improved with regular orgasms, which we can give ourselves. We'll feel better mentally and physically, and our bodies will be more resistant to illness. We'll even sleep better!

A Confession

It surprises me now that I didn't start self-pleasuring until six months after partner sex stopped. I just didn't feel the urge. I was so deeply in grief that I didn't feel capable of pleasure, and masturbation didn't seem worth the effort.

How odd for me as a sex educator to lose my sexual self that way. I knew the benefits and the importance of keeping myself sexually healthy without a partner, especially as an older person whose genitals and sexual responsiveness do not take care of themselves. If we don't keep the blood flow going to the genitals on a regular basis, we'll become less able to get aroused and reach orgasm as time goes on. I had taught exactly these concepts to others!

Grief and Masturbation

A perspective from Carlyle Jansen, sex and relationship therapist and author of **Sex Yourself**

Solo sex allows you to reconnect with and reclaim your body. It can feel awkward at first when you're in grief. You may feel guilty for having that pleasure. But your loved one would want you to live fully and to enjoy these sensations. Masturbation can help you bring yourself back into your body. It can feel freeing and helpful, even if you don't feel desire at the start.

Start by touching yourself and being mindful of engaging your nerve endings for a short period of time. Sex of any kind does not have to end in orgasm. But if you find it frustrating when an orgasm does not happen, vibrators and other sex toys are fabulous accoutrements that can make it much easier to feel heights of pleasure.

Orgasm is a release after a buildup of tension. It is often used to relieve stress and pain, and it can release grief. If you find yourself crying during solo sex, let the tears flow. Keep the stimulation going if you can, and let your pleasure clear out the stuck emotions. Masturbation is a great way to get those tears out. It is cathartic and healing in ways that can touch deeper parts of ourselves.

My Love Affair with Vibrators

I have the best unpaid job ever: I review sex toys from a senior perspective on my blog, https://joanprice.com/blog. I get to describe the qualities of exemplary sex toys that stand out in a sea of thousands. When I say I review them from a senior perspective, I mean I evaluate the ergonomic design and ease of use for creaky bodies and arthritic wrists, the intensity level for those of us with reluctant arousal, the body-safe materials so important for our health, and how easily we can use the controls without putting on our reading glasses, among other criteria. I also have the pleasure of highlighting vendors that are committed to our health and pleasure, not just sales.

Whether you're a senior or not, sex toys—particularly vibrators—can be important tools for sexual pleasure. This is especially important when you're grieving. When you're filled with sadness and loss, your body may have difficulty with arousal and orgasm. Your sensations may be dulled by depression. Your brain may not get the message that stimulation and orgasm can be a welcome relief.

During my nonsexual time after Robert's death, I didn't even look at my huge assortment of sex toys. At one point, I said to my grief counselor, "I know I should be keeping myself sexually healthy through solo pleasuring, but I'm so sad that it hardly seems worth the effort. I don't know if it would even work."

She replied with a knowing smile, "If you use a vibrator, it will work." She was right.

Vibrators can be the rescue party, increasing sexual stimulation until your brain and body come (or cum) together with pleasure and relief.

A Griever Shares

"I started out by exploring solo. When sexual feelings began to resurface after some time in my grieving process, at my therapist's suggestion, I got a new vibrator. I began by exploring my own body and seeing what that felt like. I imagined that I was with my husband again. While it made me very sad on one level, it also made me feel closer to him, as if we were continuing our relationship, only with him being on another plane of existence outside of this physical one."

"Tingle Time"

A simple way to get back to your solo sex practice (or to start one, if this is new to you) is this easy trick. For quicker, easier, and more satisfying arousal, figure out what time of day you feel most easily aroused sexually. You may not realize that your sexual responsiveness ebbs and flows during the day, and that at certain times you'll be more physically responsive and your solo sex session will feel more exciting. I call this your "tingle time." For example, many people feel that quiver of erotic possibility first thing in the morning, or after their daily dose of caffeine, or after exercise or a relaxing shower.

Try tracking your "tingle time" for a few days. Then start scheduling your solo sex time to coincide with that enhanced erotic responsiveness. You'll find you can arouse yourself and reach orgasm more easily at that time.

Don't expect that your "tingle time" will happen after a meal, when the blood flow is going to your digestive system instead of to your genitals. The timing of your medications or the challenges of your medical conditions may affect your responsiveness, also. Experiment, and enjoy the exploration.

When You've Been Taught That Masturbation Is Wrong

Younger readers may find this hard to believe, but many people of my generation were taught that masturbation was wrong. Even today, this belief persists among religions that censure sexual pleasure outside of marriage. I hear from readers all the time who are trying to unravel the influence of their early teachings. My therapist friend, the late David Pittle, PhD, MDiv, said this:

"Most of us over sixty grew up with a pile of bad teaching about masturbation: 'It will make you go blind;' 'It is prohibited by our religion;' 'Nice girls don't.' Our parents, pastors, priests and imams were wrong. Not only is masturbation not sinful, it is very healthy and contributes to our physical and mental well-being. If you are not masturbating, then you would do well to begin. Spell the word as 'Loving yourself.'

"In my practice, I find a different perspective on life between those who practice self-love and those who don't. It is certainly not an 'approved' therapy tool, but when I see someone who exhibits depression, I often ask the question, 'When was the last time you had an orgasm, either with a partner or solo?' The answer is almost always a version of 'It has been a long time.' "

How does this relate to grief? Please understand that you are a sexual being. Nurturing this part of you will help you find a release, however temporary, and will help you stay healthier physically and psychologically. You may or may not want a sex partner right now, but this self-nurturing is, if you don't mind the pun, within arm's reach.

Some Quotes to Inspire You

Here are some of my favorite quotes about solo sex:

- "We have reason to believe that man first walked upright to free his hands for masturbation."
  —Lily Tomlin

- "Among all types of sexual activity, masturbation is, however, the one in which the female most frequently reaches orgasm."
  —Alfred Charles Kinsey, *Sexual Behavior in the Human Female*, 1953

- "We know that more than 70 to 80 percent of women masturbate, and 90 percent of men masturbate, and the rest lie."
  —Joycelyn Elders, former US Surgeon General

- "How to have sex with friends, lovers, wives, husbands all begins and ends with masturbation."
  —Betty Dodson (dubbed "the Mother of Masturbation"), at age eighty-eight

- "If God didn't want us to masturbate, we wouldn't have been given these long arms."
  —Dan Savage in a *Savage Lovecast* episode

- "Remember, if you ever need a helping hand, you'll find one at the end of your arm. I really hope no one misinterprets this quote as being about masturbation."
  —Audrey Hepburn

And here's something to make you smile:

A Griever Shares

"It's been an aspect of our ongoing communication since my husband died that lights would flash or blow out oddly and appliances would turn themselves on. One year on Valentine's Day, I kept hearing an odd, muffled humming sound somewhere in my bedroom that I couldn't identify or locate. Finally, in a box next to the bed was the answer—my vibrator had turned itself on! It never had before and hasn't since. I'm sure it was my husband saying Happy Valentine's Day!"

Your Takeaway

Plan to give yourself an orgasm at least twice a week—more if you want—during your "tingle time." Then do it!

CHAPTER 5

Dating Again

"A simple equation: woman in deep grief searching for loving comfort + guys who didn't sign up for that = nobody wins. I'd spent months feeling like a taxi nobody wanted to hail."

—Rebecca Soffer in *Modern Loss: Candid Conversation about Grief. Beginners Welcome*

T here are no bad dates," I tell my "How the Heck Do I Date at This Age?" attendees, "there are only good stories." There may be tears and fears and ghosts when you start—or attempt to start—dating, but I assure you, if you keep at it, it will get better. Take every first date as an opportunity to practice dating again as you seek to resolve these quandaries:

- What kind of person am I looking for?

- What kind of relationship would work for me right now?

- How do I meet people?

- What sort of person will find me appealing?

- Can I be myself on a date or do I need to play a role?

- How much do I reveal about my grief?

- Is it off limits to talk about my deceased partner?

- What if I get rejected?

- How can I see myself with a new person when I've been with my late partner exclusively for [fill in the blank] years?

A Griever Shares

"After about three years, I thought I was ready to find someone to be with. I joined several dating sites. I thought I was ready, but I had a problem making that sexual advance. I still have that problem. Am I ready yet? I think so, I hope so, and after eight years you would think I am, but I'm still not sure."

I've learned a lot from my eleven years of not dating, dating, withdrawing from dating, dating again, not having sex, having sex, crying, laughing, and finally enjoying new partners. The emotions sometimes felt out of control, and I didn't know which "me" to present to another person when I didn't know which "me" was true or would be true the next morning.

If you don't know if you're ready to date, it's okay to try it and then put dating on hold if it feels wrong. You're not making any kind of commitment that you can't reverse. The same is true for sex. You can explore, then change your mind at any point.

"Don't be surprised to experience any of these when you're starting to date again: massive panic, fear of rejection, renewed grief and guilt over moving on, exasperation when your date doesn't measure up to your deceased partner. These are all common reactions. You'll feel both giddy and scared, elated and disappointed. Expect an emotional roller coaster. This is one reason to go slowly. Avoid committing long hours with someone new. Understand that after a while, you'll adjust, and these upsetting feelings will calm down. Try the toe-dipping scenario: try it, back off, try it again. Take your time, go slowly, be in a learning mode."

—Tina B. Tessina, PhD, "Dr. Romance," psychotherapist, author of *Dr. Romance's Guide to Finding Love Today*

How Do I Meet People?

There are basically two ways to meet potential dates:

1. **Get out socially.** Do the activities you enjoy and try new activities that appeal to you. You'll meet others who have interests in common. Advantage: If you don't meet someone, you'll still enjoy what you're doing. Disadvantage: Even if you meet people who attract you, you have no idea

whether they're available or interested in dating you.

2. **Use online dating.** That's where the people are who are looking to date. Advantage: You can see their photos and read their profiles before choosing whom to meet. Disadvantage: There's a learning curve if you've never done it before, and it can be time-consuming and discouraging to wade through the people who are not right for you as you try to find the ones who are.

I suggest you do both. When I teach my "How the Heck Do I Date at This Age?" workshop and recommend online dating, some people are dismayed. "Oh, no," they tell me. "I'm not going to get involved in that." But think of it this way: If people who would be a good match for you are trying to find you, where would they go? They wouldn't go searching coffee shops in your town at the same moment you're sitting there waiting. No, they'd join an online dating site and hope you find each other. Give it a chance for three or six months. Ask an experienced friend who knows you well to help you with your profile.

If you're in my age group, or even if you're not, I hope you'll consider watching my webinar, "How the Heck Do I Date at This Age?" or attending live if I give this workshop near you. I developed this workshop in early 2012, after fumbling through this process and emerging with plenty of useful information, tips, and attitude adjustments that could help others. In it, I give a complete road map to meeting people, online dating, writing a good profile, first dates, moving toward sex, and so much more. You don't have to reinvent the wheel!

A Griever Shares

"Relatively new to my area with limited contacts and no prospects, I decided to try online dating. After one first date that extended from coffee into a few hours of conversation, I was exhilarated that I could meet a nice guy, share my story without breaking down, and mildly enjoy the company of a man who was not the one who had been at my side for thirty-eight years. I felt a spark of physical attraction and longing. Hello, long-lost libido!"

Try Not to Compare

If your relationship with your beloved was a good one, you can't help comparing the new people you meet with an idealized version of your lost partner. It's natural, but it's not the best way to give new people a chance. Instead of mentally listing the many ways your new date falls short compared to your beloved, try to get interested in the new human beings you meet on their own terms. This isn't an interview for the job of "next long-term partner"—it's only an interview for the next date.

Let each first and next date be an opportunity to learn more about yourself as well as about your date. For example,

- What can I learn about this new person?

- What questions can I ask that elicit interesting answers?

- What do I feel comfortable revealing about myself?

- What am I learning from this date about the kind of person I'm looking for?

- What am I learning about how to have a dialogue with a stranger?

- What am I learning about myself from this date?

A Griever Shares

"I missed male companionship, so about a year after my husband died, I went online to look at the pool of lonely gentlemen in my age group. 'Friends first, then see what develops' seemed to be a common theme in many of the men's profile narratives. 'Chemistry' was another criterion. When I looked at a picture of a man in the online profiles, I asked myself, 'Could I see myself making love with this man?' I couldn't help comparing each of them with my late husband. None seemed to be his match."

Should You Only Date Widows/Widowers/Grievers?

When I wrote my first online dating profile after Robert died, I specified that I was looking to date a widower. After all, who else could understand what I was going through? Who else would understand the depth of losing the most important person in my life and the moxie it took to start dating again?

Indeed, my dates with widowers were satisfying because we had that commonality of experience. We understood how each other's worlds were permanently altered because our beloveds had been ripped from us. We noticed but didn't correct each other when one of us lapsed into present tense when talking about the deceased partner. We were able to have vulnerable conversations within minutes of meeting each other. We were compassionate when laughter turned into tears. We understood the need for silences in our conversation.

Later, with more years of dating behind me, I saw some disadvantages of dating only people who had lost their beloveds:

- It restricts the dating pool too much if you're not in a city of size.

- Your date may be too raw or miserable to have much to give.

- Just because you have grief in common doesn't mean you have anything else in common. (How often I experienced this!)

Eleven years after Robert's death and with an array of dating experiences under my belt, I still think that dating someone who knows grief is helpful. I'm dating a widower now. Being able to share our grief stories spontaneously has intensified our intimacy. We know how to listen to each other's anecdotes and respond to each other's feelings with compassion and understanding. We feel heard, understood, accepted.

A Griever Shares

"My grief is often suppressed and below the
level of consciousness until, suddenly and
unexpectedly, it's triggered by a place, a song, or
a memory, and I'm reduced to tears. Despite my
grief, about a month after my wife died, I joined
OkCupid. I had face-to-face meetings with more
than half a dozen women. I met three of these for
a second date, and I continue to see one woman
regularly more than a year and a half after our
memorable first date. She is also widowed,
and we each continue to grieve the loss of our
beloveds. We share our grief experiences with
each other and move onward with our lives. For
me, dating while grieving has been essential to
my ability to recover and move forward."

Moving Gradually toward Sex

You may want to explore kissing or tentative
touching with your date before you're fully ready
for a sexual relationship. The first time I let

myself enjoy a long, soulful kiss with a new man, I was amazed to feel aroused. I loved feeling those tingly sensations running through my body as the kissing continued. We didn't take it past kissing then (though we did eventually), and that didn't matter. It was a way for the two of us to explore, "Are we attracted to each other?" and for me to discover, "Hallelujah, I feel sexy sparks again!"

If you sense that your date is expecting that these first explorations will lead to shedding clothes and heading for bed, it's a good idea to set boundaries verbally. You'd like to do X right now and set the limits at Y. Define those your own way. For example:

- "I'm enjoying our kissing, and that's as far as I want to go tonight."

- "This feels wonderful, but let's stop here."

- "I feel vulnerable and need to know we can stop when I want."

A Griever Shares

"Widowed at fifty-five, I felt grief and extreme loneliness. I also felt a surge in my sexual feelings, which was disturbing. Three months after my wife died, I decided to go on a dating site. Living in England and being a bit of a swivel-eyed leftie, the Guardian newspaper's dating site seemed a natural choice. An older widow wished to meet, 'if only to share experiences of being bereaved.' We engaged in a frenetic exchange of emails: twenty-six in four days! We bared our souls and reminisced about the wonderful spouses we had lost.

"When we did meet, she was reserved. I was sexually attracted to her and wanted to snuggle up to her, but she wasn't ready for that, and we parted awkwardly. She emailed that she didn't feel she could have me as a lover. I spent the weekend feeling like a dumped teenager.

"Then she emailed to say that she couldn't get me out of her mind. She invited me to her house, where we hugged and kissed. We didn't have sex, but it didn't matter. I was so happy that we were together for that evening, and I made my way home, light-headed as a teenager who had just snogged the girl he'd been lusting after for months. The next day she emailed to say she wanted me to 'take the lead physically.' Wow, the stuff of an adolescent boy's dreams: a lovely older woman who offers her body to me without my even having to ask her."

Your Takeaway

Make a list of what you do and don't want when your first or next date happens. Rehearse asking for what you want and communicating boundaries. Revise this list and rehearse the communication before each new date until you feel grounded and in control.

CHAPTER 6

For Non-Grievers Who Want to Date Us

"Death ends a life, but it does not end a relationship, and survivors often struggle to resolve what seems like an unresolvable contradiction. We need to have a better understanding of our capacity as human beings to have multiple relationships, to hold both past and present loves within ourselves at once."

—Julia Samuel, in *Grief Works: Stories of Life, Death, and Surviving*

U nderstand that you're not in competition with your griever's deceased partner. You're not the "replacement" lover. What you share with the griever you're dating is an entirely new relationship. You both come to each other with your history, your experiences, your past lovers.

A Griever Shares

"Our relationships with our deceased beloveds endure beyond their death, and any non-griever who wishes to date us needs to comprehend this. Our past loves remain an integral part of us even as we seek to create new present loves. Non-grievers who don't grasp this won't 'get' us, and any relationship they wish to have with us probably is doomed to failure."

I received this email from a non-griever:

I have dated many widows, and their reactions are varied:

1. I find it really difficult to be invited to the home of a lady and find she's turned it into a shrine to her late husband.

2. Some ladies really want to enjoy sex again, but it bothers them that it's not "him" and they can't achieve orgasm, despite my best loving efforts.

3. A few feel *free* and have no problem diving back into the dating game and enjoy having a healthy sex life again.

All of these are natural responses, and this is true for any gender, not just widows. We all respond sexually to a new person on our own timetable, which is not within our control. This non-griever seems compassionate about numbers 2 and 3, but perhaps judgmental about number 1. Or maybe I'm reading it that way because I'm feeling defensive personally. Here's why:

Who Defines "Shrine"?

You could say that my house is a shrine to my late husband, though I don't really see it that way. Robert Rice was an extraordinary artist, and thirty-six of his paintings hang in my house. Seven are in my bedroom. He was also a dancer, and his dance shoes still have a spot in my dance room, along with a heart he painted with the penciled words, "Dancing with you." Photos are here and there through the house—no longer in the bedroom, but you can't walk through any other room without seeing him dancing or painting or holding me. These photos and paintings do not make me sad—they're part of my life. I wouldn't want to date someone who thought I should put them away.

But that's me. You may feel different. If you are dating a griever, I understand that once your relationship progresses to the bedroom, your sexual energy might be deflated by finding yourself face-to-face with a wedding photo. Instead of suggesting changes in the bedroom décor, though, how about inviting your date to your house instead, or to a hotel, if that's in your budget? Having sex in a place that doesn't hold old memories could be good emotionally for your date as well as for you, but that's a decision the two of you should make.

In my view, it's fine to say, "I'd feel more comfortable being sexual with you in a neutral place that doesn't hold all these visual memories. Would you be open to coming to my house when we want to be intimate?" It's not okay to say, "I need you to remove your partner's photos now that we're together."

I preface that with "in my view," because we all grieve differently, and we all get ready for sex with a new person differently. The email writer above has experienced three drastically different ways that widows experience dating a new person—you may have additional experiences. No one is doing grief "wrong."

"It would be great if people came with care instructions: When I feel sad, please do this. You'll know to back off when you see me do or say these things...We can get better at hearing what others need by practicing attention and open communication throughout our lives, across all of our relationships."

—Megan Devine in *It's OK that You're Not OK: Meeting Grief and Loss in a Culture that Doesn't Understand*

Tips for Dating Someone Who Has Lost a Partner

You'll need to talk with the person you're dating. Don't avoid talking about your date's loss—that won't help either of you. As with every relationship, communication is crucial. You might start by going over the tips below. Which ones resonate with your griever? With you? What would you change or add? This conversation isn't just an icebreaker. It may be a way to cut through the chatter and the silence and get deep.

Do: Ask how best to support them when grief hits, because it will.

Don't: Assume you know. Even if you've dated other grievers, you don't know what *this* griever needs.

"Grieving people would much rather have you stumble through your acts of bearing witness than have you confidently assert that things are not as bad as they seem. You can't always change pain, but you can change how you hear pain, how you respond to pain. When pain exists, let it exist. Bear witness. Make it safe for the other to say, 'This hurts,' without rushing in to clean it up."

—Megan Devine in *It's OK that You're Not OK: Meeting Grief and Loss in a Culture that Doesn't Understand*

Do: Understand if tears come when they talk about their partner. Or even for no reason. Keep listening through the tears.

Don't: Try to fix their grief or make it better. You can't, and it will just make things worse.

A Griever Shares

"Have patience. Be a listener. Support the griever's feelings and give them the space they need."

Do: Listen to stories about the deceased and their relationship.

Don't: Date someone who's grieving if you don't feel comfortable hearing stories about the person who died.

> ### A Griever Shares
>
> "Ask about their spouse or partner who has passed on. Don't be shy about it. Chances are they will be happy to share memories and stories. I love to talk about my darling husband. You will get a window into what makes that person happy."

Do: Get out of the house (your house, your date's house) and go somewhere new to create romantic experiences together.

Don't: Expect that your date's home is where sex with you will happen (unless invited).

Do: Consult your date about plans.

Don't: Surprise your date with an activity or destination. You may think you know the ideal spot for a romantic evening, but what if that's a special place they last visited with their partner?

Do: Take your cues for sex from the griever.

Don't: Have a goal or timetable for how or when sex happens.

A Griever Shares

"Grief is a process that has its own timeline. Never, never say to someone in grief, 'When are you going to get over it?' It is likely that I will never 'get over it.' It has become part and parcel of who I am. Don't presume to know how I should engage with my grief. You can, however, be supportive, sympathetic, and empathetic."

Do: Take sex in stages.

Don't: Assume that the first sexual exploration needs to have any specific activity or outcome.

(See Chapters 8, **Your (New) First Time**, and 9, **It's Not All or Nothing**.)

Do: Respond compassionately if sex starts and it doesn't work for the griever. Gently ask what they're feeling and what they're willing to share about what happened.

Don't: Press for details if they can't or won't talk about it, and don't judge the griever for not being ready.

Do: Understand that there can be room for you *and* the deceased in your griever's heart.

Don't: Feel you're competing with the deceased for the griever's affection, attention, or love.

A Griever Shares

"For non-grievers who are dating someone who is grieving, remember that when we speak with love and affection and longing about our deceased partners, it is in no way a commentary on how we feel about our new partners."

You may discover you're not the right fit for this person at this time, or maybe ever. Most new relationships don't work out, whether the problems have to do with grief or not. But don't dismiss someone with whom there's chemistry, compatibility, and interest just because *you* think grief is a problem. Give the relationship a chance to blossom.

Your Takeaway

If you're a griever, what other tips would you suggest to someone who wants to date you? If you're dating a griever, what do you know now that you wish you had known earlier? Email joan@joanprice.com, and I'll create a blog post with these tips.

CHAPTER 7

It's Okay If You're Not Ready

"I still miss him so much that I dissolve in tears and gut-wrenching sadness. Then a few minutes later, I'm thinking it's time for my lips to be kissed and my breasts to be touched."

—From Joan's Grief Journal, Sept. 2010

Two months after the above journal entry, and one and a half years after Robert's death, I shared this on my blog:

> I had a "date" with a man with whom I had shared an intensely sensual relationship twenty-seven years before, when I was forty and he (get ready) was twenty-three. We had enjoyed each other immensely, then both of us

had gone on to other relationships, and he had moved many states away.

Suddenly we discovered that we would be in the same city last Saturday. With anticipation and fantasies abounding, we arranged to meet. How lovely, I daydreamed. Here's a smart, gentle, witty man from my past who gloried in giving me pleasure, and we were always able to talk candidly. Surely the twenty-seven years apart could be wiped out for an evening of sensual nostalgia, couldn't it? I needed to rise from grief and rediscover my sensuality with a live person rather than with sex toys. This sweet man could be the one to take my hand and lead me there.

We met, we hugged, we talked excitedly about where our lives and loves had taken us in the past decades. But then, when the time came to kiss and discover, I couldn't. I felt myself sinking into sadness. His kiss wasn't Robert's. His body type wasn't Robert's. I pulled away.

"I really hoped I would respond sexually to you," I told him, "but I'm not."

"I'm sorry," he said, cradling my head against his chest.

"I even packed condoms and lubricant, and chose my underwear with care," I added. He laughed with me at that last revelation. "But it's just not happening. I still miss Robert so much."

"Tell me about him," he said, maybe the sweetest comment he could have made.

I waited another two years before having intercourse with a new partner. This surprises me. I hadn't realized it was that long, but my journal doesn't lie. This man was a trusted friend who had been an occasional sex buddy for a couple of years before Robert. He was a generous lover, but although my body responded, I fought back tears. I wrote in my journal, "Although I'm ready to be there, I'm not there." It would be another year and a half before I could respond fully with another partner, who became a regular "friend with benefits." (See Chapter 11, **Friends with Benefits**.)

No Shame, No Judgment

A well-meaning friend told me, "I'm worried that you're stuck." I don't remember if it was two or four years after Robert's death, but that doesn't matter. What matters is that my personal timetable was right for me. I was moving through grief at my own pace, and it was irrelevant whether I adhered to some external schedule for when I "should" be ready to have partner sex again.

The decision to invite a new person into your bed may feel incredibly complicated. I yearned for touch and sex, but I couldn't transfer those feelings from missing Robert's touch to wanting a new man's touch. You may vacillate, as I did. The desire for sex and the retreat from sex may coexist. Whatever you do or don't do, I encourage you to see it all as a healthy process. It's okay to explore getting close to a new lover and then change your mind.

As always, honesty is good—both with yourself and with a potential new lover. Someone who doesn't get your grief isn't right for you at this time.

I've heard about breakups, "The best way to get over someone is to get under someone else," but this isn't a breakup. You're not trying to wrench your heart free from your beloved—you're trying to reconcile your loss with your own life force. That can take time.

A Griever Shares

"I'm still figuring out what kind of sex I'm willing to do, and yet wanting to find another woman to be with. My stages have been 1. Loneliness; 2. Guilt; 3. Sex with loneliness and guilt and lots of masturbating; 4. Dating with lots of masturbating while hoping to find a partner."

Cycling through Healing

A perspective from Tina B. Tessina, PhD, "Dr. Romance," psychotherapist, author of **Dr. Romance's Guide to Finding Love Today**

Grief is multi-faceted: It includes sadness, anger, fear, silliness, fond memories, tears, and numbness. You will cycle through all of these. Grief can blindside you when you thought you were mostly through it; it can be because of some little reminder, or a significant calendar date, or something someone says that reminds you of your lost love. Every new step in a new relationship will remind you of your lost one. All these feelings are part of your healing, and they will come and go. Your sexual feelings will be affected by your grief, so they will swirl around in the same way.

Do your best to just be with whatever is going on. Give yourself alone time when you need it, time to write, and someone to talk to about all these feelings. If you are open about your feelings of grief, your sexual energy will revive. Sharing grief is creating intimacy, and intimacy leads to sexual feelings.

If You Think It's Too Soon for Sex with a New Partner, It Is

Your body, your brain, and your spirit need to align so that sex is good. It may take one year, or five, or, as Lynn Brown Rosenberg, author of *My Sexual Awakening at 70*, describes, it may take twelve years:

> Mine was a long road back to sex after losing my husband, but oh, boy, when it came back, it came with a vengeance! For the first several years I didn't want to get close to anyone. I sought help and medication for depression from a psychiatrist. I joined a grief group. Nothing could get me over the hump.

> Twelve long years passed without sex. Finally, I told my doctor, "It's been a long time since I had an orgasm."

She said, "Get some porn and a vibrator." I did exactly what she said and started having orgasms like crazy.

I eventually realized that I had been sexually repressed and didn't want to be that way anymore. I talked to men on sex sites, I watched porn on the Internet. Then I had sex with real people. It was opening and freeing.

Your Takeaway

Don't judge yourself if you're not ready. Everyone progresses at a different speed. Don't let anyone rush you. Meanwhile, keep yourself sexually healthy with your own hands and sex toys.

CHAPTER 8

Your (New) First Time

You know it will happen. This person is charming and attractive and makes you laugh. You feel comfortable together. The chemistry between you is intense. You've talked, kissed, and made a date that you know, hope, or fantasize will be sexual. Who knew it was possible to feel like a teenager again? You're so excited—this will be wonderful.

Or...

You're nervous, self-conscious, and ambivalent. What if you can't go through with it? Your new partner won't find your old, naked body desirable. You won't know how to satisfy this stranger. What if you're too embarrassed and sad to enjoy it? How will you handle it if the sex turns out to be mediocre, not satisfying, or a disaster? What if you cry?

Although there's no magic formula to make sure your (new) first time is closer to the first example than the second, there are ways you can improve your chances:

- **Face your fears.** Figure out what's driving your ambivalence: Body image? Sexual skill? Fear of bursting into tears? Not trusting your new partner? Not feeling ready? Talk this over with a counselor or a wise, trusted friend.

- **Practice asking for what you want.** You spent years with your beloved, and you learned to please each other and read each other's cues and subtleties. We're all different, and a new person cannot possibly know what *you* need and desire unless you learn how to communicate it.

- **Set boundaries for your first time.** Realize that you can get sexual in stages (please read the next chapter, **It's Not All or Nothing**). Make sure your partner agrees to observe the boundaries you set.

- **Find your voice.** Communicate to your new partner before, during, and after your sex date. Don't "hint": say it clearly and kindly. If you don't feel you can talk candidly, reconsider whether this is the right person for you in your vulnerability.

A Griever Shares

"You would think, that, in her sixties, a woman could be herself with confidence and verve, and just go for it. But, no, the insecure, inexperienced young woman was still inside. Over the decades of building our relationship, my husband gave me a lot of feedback and interaction that built my self-confidence. I learned so much from him and our interactions about love, trust, and sex. It was always an adventure with him."

Navigating Your First Time

A perspective from Stella Harris, sex coach, author of **Tongue Tied: Untangling Communication in Sex, Kink, and Relationships**

Grief can be a whole mind and body experience, and heartache affects the brain just like physical pain. It's difficult to predict how that will affect your arousal patterns and your orgasm. Having sex, partnered or solo, can be part of the healing process.

Before sex for the first time with someone new, explain your situation. It's okay to say, "I might cry." Let them know what you'd like them to do if that happens. Do you want to keep going, just feeling your feelings? Or do you want to stop if tears come?

Physical arousal—the way your genitals respond—does not always align with mental arousal. Your mind might be interested but your body may not respond, or you might feel physical arousal when you aren't mentally ready. If your mind is ready when your body isn't, try easing into things. What steps toward intimate or sensual pleasures can you explore? Our bodies learn pleasure the way our muscles learn tasks, and they can get out of practice. You may need to show your body the way back when it's time.

If you have a sexual encounter without orgasm, that's okay. It's not failed sex—it's successful intimacy. Not every encounter leads to orgasm, under any circumstances. Try not to add blame or shame to the already difficult feelings you're experiencing. You might tell your partner in advance that you're not sure if you'll have an orgasm, but that you'd like to explore touch and pleasure anyway.

Taking a new lover isn't replacing the person you lost, it's simply continuing your own journey of growth and self-discovery. There's no "right" amount of time to wait before you try to experience romance or sex again. And sometimes you won't know you're ready until you try.

Use Your Words

I keep emphasizing the need for clear communication. I know this is difficult for many of us, especially after we're used to being understood by a longtime partner without having to explain much. Assume that your new partner wants very much to please you but is bad at reading your mind. It's a gift to help your partner by being clear.

No two bodies respond to the same stimulus in the same way. Our emotional responses are also unique. And as we know, grief clouds everything that used to be normal. So how can a new partner—a stranger to your body and your pleasures and desires—know how to please you without some help from you? As a former lover said to me, "I love it when you give me directions, so I know I'm doing what you like."

I don't mean that you should print out a step-by-step instruction manual with diagrams. But do give gentle guidance and ask for the same from your partner. For example:

- "I like it when you..."

- "I'd like you to..."

- "I like to be touched this way..."

- "Oh, that's nice!"

- "Let's just do this for now..."

- "Do you like...?"

- "What would you enjoy?"

A Griever Shares

"My insecurity is probably off the charts. I knew what and how to please my wife. I loved trying to make her happy during sex. But what another woman likes or doesn't like is completely foreign to me. I have tried, often feeling like I was failing. I think I need better communication, but I don't want to offend or take anything for granted. I just don't know what I'm doing. I think I need a partner to be assertive, take the lead, and let me know what to do, what she likes, and how I can please her."

When New Sex Doesn't Satisfy

You've fantasized about sex with this new person, and you're ready. You anticipate letting that built-up horniness soar and release, thanks to the capable hands, mouth, and genitals of your new lover. And then, boom, letdown. You're left disappointed and sadder than before. One or more of these issues may be causing this:

- Your new lover isn't your former partner, and you're in grief. You'd give anything to be making love with your beloved instead of this semi-stranger in bed with you.

- You feel guilty, as if you're cheating on your deceased partner. (You're not.)

- You feel insecure about your body, your desirability, your sexual skills. Concentrate on the connection and the pleasure instead of judging yourself.

- Your new partner doesn't know you and doesn't know what you like, how to please you, what turns you on, what gets you off. (See **Use Your Words** above.)

- Your new lover just isn't the right person for you. That's okay—move on in your search for someone who's better for you.

- It's too soon. You thought it was time, but it's not.

A Griever Shares

"I met my husband at eighteen when I was a virgin. We were together forty-one years, and he was my only sexual experience. We grew and learned what worked for us along the way. I was happy having screaming, multiple orgasms. After his death, I was so horny, pleasuring myself to get relief. After two years. I joined dating sites and felt a crazy connection with a new man. I was so nervous the first time we had sex, but wildly excited to have a real penis! The sex wasn't great. He wasn't like my husband. He didn't know how to please me. We talked about things I liked ahead of time, but maybe he just wasn't that good."

Many Grievers Share

I received so many responses to this topic! Here's what grievers shared about their (new) first times. They had good times. They had bad times. They struggled with all the challenges above, the same insecurities that you face. The variety helps affirm that whatever your experience is, you're not alone.

"That first partnered sex after such a long hiatus opened a floodgate of emotions. I found it spectacular and reaffirming that at my age, and as a widower, I could still be attractive to someone."

*

"I was widowed seven years ago at the age of fifty-four. After his death, I felt sexually dormant for at least a year and totally lacked desire. Gradually, my loneliness compelled me to start looking for a new relationship, though the thought of being physically intimate was intimidating and terrifying. The idea of being naked with someone who would know my body with all its wear and tear was difficult to imagine, much less anticipate as pleasurable. I guess I was hoping for a guy whose ultimate fantasy was a woman in floor-length flannel that he discovered only in pitch blackness!"

*

"After a forty-three-year relationship with my husband being my one and only, I felt insecure about initiating a sexual relationship with another man. I felt like an awkward teenager. Am I attractive enough? Am I too fat? Do I look repulsive naked? How do I initiate intimacy? What signals am I sending? Do I make a move and kiss him first? Will I be rejected or embraced? Will I look too desperate, too needy? How do I even touch a man? What's right and what's wrong? What will please him or repulse him? Do I just ask?"

*

"I am a sixty-six-year-old widower after a thirty-eight-year marriage. My first sexual experience about six months after my wife passed was a nightmare. I was extremely lonely, so I joined a dating site. A woman in my town responded and wanted to get to know me. We met at a local park, we talked, then she kissed me. I thought, wow, I'm so lucky to have found someone who understands and wants to be with me. We went to her house, where we were intimate. She took control and I gladly did anything she asked, just to be with someone. When I got home, my guilt was overwhelming. I felt like I had cheated on my wife. I quit the dating site, told her I couldn't see her again, and I didn't date again for three years. Dating is hard. I was never unfaithful to my wife, and now I fight with my feelings of guilt, that I'm somehow cheating on her. I know I'm not, but I often feel like I am."

*

"The guys brag about how good they are at pleasing women, but I haven't experienced it. I explained that I have a hard time having orgasm with just penetration. I have great orgasms with oral sex. The guys would say they were good at oral sex and liked it. But they would be down there for only a minute or two and forget that I needed that for orgasms. I've only been trying to date for the last seven months now. I am not enjoying it. I really miss the comfort of my husband."

*

"I was terrified of taking that step toward intimacy after I started dating a woman several years after my wife died, so we took it very slowly. The first few times, we just used our hands to pleasure each other in the car after a date, which made me feel like a teenager again. Finally, one day my girlfriend asked for help moving a piece of furniture. When I entered her house, she was wearing only a bra and panties. Because we had already learned to pleasure each other and we went at a comfortable pace, the first time was wonderful. We missed our dinner reservation and stayed in bed together all night. It was strange to me being with someone new who liked different things and dealing with condoms for the first time in thirty-some years. But that also made it very exciting for me."

*

"I did feel a little awkward about enjoying sex so much with someone new, but my wife and I had agreed years before that if either of us were to die, the other should feel no qualms about finding solace in the arms of someone new."

Safer Sex

Please use safer sex protection with every sex partner, at every sexual encounter—no exceptions. I could scare you with the STI statistics in the over-fifty population, or I could entice you with how much fun condoms can be in sex play. I've written widely about safer sex in my books and articles, and I've made a forty-five-minute YouTube video—"Safer Sex for Seniors with Joan Price"—which you can watch for free. Please watch that video before you have oral or penetrative sex with your next partner. It will help you see that safer sex can be fun and erotic whatever your age—and it is necessary.

For More

If you're in my age group, or even if you're not, I hope you'll read the two chapters titled "Sex with a New Partner" and "Safer Sex Always" in *The Ultimate Guide to Sex after 50: How to Maintain—or Regain!—a Spicy, Satisfying Sex Life*. I can't distill all the information and tips from those forty-two pages into a few pages here, and there's so much in those chapters that is relevant to getting sexual after grief.

Your Takeaway

Write down the points you'll want to bring up when you decide to have sex with a new person: what you do and don't want, the pace that will make you comfortable, any concerns you'll want to share. Practice a future conversation so it will be easier when it happens.

It's Not All or Nothing

"Sex is a lot like a buffet. We have so many
different choices for pleasure and intimacy.
Intercourse is a popular dish, and it's a favorite
for many people. But there's no reason to skip
past all the other options or consider them only
as appetizers. When you do that, you miss out on
discovering lots of other delicious possibilities!"

**—Charlie Glickman, PhD, sex and relationship
coach, www.makesexeasy.com.**

B y seeing penetrative sex as the primary
goal, those of us with penises (and those
of us who have sex with people with penises)
cheat ourselves out of a lot of sexual pleasure.
Heterosexual couples especially tend to fall into
this pattern: we're turned on, we arouse each
other, we finish with intercourse, aka PIV (penis-
in-vagina). This is the old model, and it's limiting
for several reasons:

- As grievers, we may be ready for sexual touch and sexual release long before we're ready for penetrative sex.

- Older vulva owners may experience vaginal discomfort with PIV, especially if it's been a long time since penetrative sex. This can cause anxiety and sometimes avoidance of sex. What if my vagina won't comfortably receive his penis? What if extended intercourse will cause me vaginal pain?

- Older penis owners may have difficulty achieving and maintaining erections for intercourse. This can cause performance anxiety. What if I can't get hard enough for penetration? What if I can't stay hard for the length of time it takes to reach orgasm?

- Since 75 percent of vulva owners do **not** reach orgasm solely through intercourse, why is PIV the goal anyway?

- Intercourse is only one of the many ways we can enjoy sex and reach orgasm.

- Our skin is our largest sex organ. Our bodies
  are wonderlands of sensation. Seeing sexual
  expression as solely one set of genitals
  entering another set of genitals limits the
  possibilities of sex.

What if we choose to experience sexual
expression without any goals except pleasure?
Imagine how freeing this can be!

When I was getting ready emotionally for sex
with a new partner, what I imagined wasn't
PIV. I fantasized about opening gradually to a
new lover through skin connection, a stranger's
hand exciting me, the surprises of new and
unpredictable touch, an orgasm that I could relax
into instead of working for it. That's the reason I
bought myself an erotic massage as my gateway
drug to becoming sexual again. (See Chapter 13,
Massage or More?)

As the years went on, I had sex with different
partners. When I say, "had sex," I mean we
aroused each other, enjoyed each other, and gave

each other orgasms. Sometimes this included PIV, and often it didn't.

A Griever Shares

"Starting over with a new sexual relationship at age sixty-three seemed daunting. So getting sexual by stages made a lot of sense and seemed the 'natural' way to go about it. Just like in teenagerhood, we are discovering a lot of things about ourselves, and learning how to act and behave in the world."

"I'm Not Sure I Can"

After I resumed sex with new partners, one of my intimate dates was a man about seventy who had recently ended an almost sexless dating relationship. On our third date (no, that's not a magic number—it just happened that way), we met at his house. We enjoyed a leisurely afternoon that included a hike, lots of talking, and then returning to his house. We held each other and kissed, and when the touching got exciting and clothes seemed superfluous, we moved to his bedroom.

I was prepared that this might happen, so I showed my date a special pouch I had brought with me. "I'd like to show you what I brought, in case we need them," I said, pulling out a packet of Überlube lubricant and a condom. I wanted him to know that I needed lubricant for any intimate touching and that my policy was safer sex, if we got to that point. I preferred an awkward conversation now to surprising him later by fumbling for these items without earlier discussion.

My date's exuberance, as well as his erection, fell. "I don't know if I can stay hard with a condom," he said. I assured him that we had no goals except pleasure. To prove it, I asked him to receive a sensual massage. When he apologized for his lack of erection, I said, "That doesn't matter. What matters is whether you're enjoying the sensation. Are you?"

"Oh, yes," he replied, and relaxed into receiving pleasure with a happy ending. Afterwards he returned the favor. We never did get to PIV, and neither of us felt deprived. The relationship wasn't sustainable—we lived too far apart, and he wasn't over his previous relationship. But it allowed me to give and receive sexual pleasure with a man who excited me.

A Griever Shares

"One of my concerns about dating was how to manage the level of physical intimacy gradually, without my date expecting that any sexual activity would culminate in intercourse. I was able to haltingly express my willingness for some but not all levels of intimacy, and he was amenable. I was surprised to find myself enjoying 'petting' sessions with the ardor of a teenager. After about six weeks, it was I who took his hand to lead him into the bedroom."

One Slow Step at a Time

I'm not saying you should deny yourself PIV if that's what you enjoy. Just don't sprint to the finish line when you're first exploring sex with a new person. Find out what kinds of touch turn your new partner on, and let your new partner learn what turns you on. Tell your partner what you do and don't want. For example, you might say,

- "Can we just kiss for now?"

- "I'd like to explore touching but no penetration."

- "My feelings are fragile, and, if we get started, I need it to be okay that I might change my mind and to know that you'll accept that."

A Griever Shares

"I wasn't sure I was ready when I started dating my boyfriend. The idea of having sex with someone else after more than twenty-three years with my husband seemed foreign and almost wrong. But this new man was someone I knew and respected, and the chemistry between us was impossible to ignore. We took our entire relationship a step at a time. He let me put the brakes on whenever I needed to. We took things as slowly as I wanted. There's not much slow about us now!"

Expanding Sex Without Penetration

I wrote "A Senior's Guide to Sex Without Intercourse" for SeniorPlanet.org in November 2016 (https://seniorplanet.org/a-seniors-guide-to-sex-without-intercourse). JP Pritchett, owner of The Smitten Kitten—an extraordinary sex toy store and educational resource in Minneapolis—told me I should turn that article into a workshop. I did, and "Great Sex Without Penetration" has become the most popular workshop I present at The Smitten Kitten and elsewhere. It's also available now as a webinar which you can find online at https://joanprice.com/webinars.

People come into the workshop feeling deflated because, for one reason or another, penetrative sex is not possible or desired. They think that this limits or even cancels their sexual expression. They leave the workshop smiling and expectant, eager to try the many suggestions I offer. Here's a quick summary of some of these tips—read the article cited above or view the webinar for full explanations.

- **Explore each other's entire bodies.** Our skin is our largest sex organ. Invite your partner to touch your body all over—no goals, just pleasure.

- **Share sensual, full-body massage.** Use a nice massage oil and take plenty of time massaging your partner's whole body. Your goal is to give delicious, relaxing pleasure.

- **Explore new erogenous zones.** Our erogenous zones can change as we age. The way to discover what turns you on now is to let go of the notions of where you're "supposed" to feel stimulation and, instead, try touching new spots to see how you respond.

- **Explore new ways to touch.** Lighter or harder, faster or slower, direct or teasing. Sometimes the difference between getting aroused or not is not *where* you touch as much as *how* you touch.

- **Use your mouth.** Oral sex rules! All genders may find that the combination of the warmth, pressure, and wetness of the mouth together with the movement of the tongue invites us to orgasm better than penetrative sex.

- **Use your hands.** Especially after plenty of all-over touching, stimulating the vulva or penis with hands and fingers can bring you to a strong orgasm. We may call them "hand jobs," but I prefer to think of this practice as "hand joys."

- **Use sex toys.** The right vibrator will help you reach orgasm, whether you're trying to stimulate a vulva or a penis. I can't stress enough how powerful these arousal tools are. (See Chapter 4, **Solo Sex**, and my webinar, "Sex Toys for Seniors.")

A Griever Shares

"My date told me there was a 'problem' with sex that we needed to discuss. Penetration was painful for her. I had fingers, lips, and a tongue as well as a penis, so we went to bed. I was amazed by the strength of her libido. We had no problem arousing each other, and, despite what she had said earlier, she said she wanted penetrative sex. We tried unsuccessfully and rather clumsily to achieve this. Then we laughed our heads off about the whole thing. It was that laughter about sexual difficulties that was just what we needed. Suddenly I could see that sex in later life could have a whole new dimension—in which we didn't need to worry about our body parts performing 'properly.' With this realization, I was able to enjoy our blissful naked embrace, even so soon after my bereavement."

Your Takeaway

Practice the conversation you might have with a new partner about getting sexual in stages. Don't worry about sexual partners being disappointed—they might be relieved.

CHAPTER 10

The Pilot Light Lover

"The Pilot Light Lover, a transitional figure...
reignites a midlife woman's capacity for love and
sex.... The Pilot Light Lover rarely lasts. He may be
a married man disguised as a single, or a great
lover but unsuitable life partner—but so what?
After the heartache wears off, a woman who is on
her way to becoming seasoned should be able to
celebrate the Pilot Light Lover's role in her journey."

**—Gail Sheehy, in *Sex and the Seasoned
Woman: Pursuing the Passionate Life***

Although Sheehy was writing specifically
for midlife women, this concept applies to
any gender at any age and is especially applicable
to people in grief. "The Pilot Light Lover" is the
person who lights up your sexual arousal and
takes your body from icy numbness to fiery
excitement. This may become a relationship
that lasts, but it's usually temporary, and that

doesn't matter. What does matter is finally being able to open your mind and body to the sweep of excitement of a new person touching you sexually.

The Pilot Light Lover's immediate gift is the tingle of sexual arousal, the feel of skin on skin, hands exploring, genitals anticipating and accepting, building into an orgasm that you and your sex toys didn't induce on your own.

Finding Your Pilot Light Lover

I hear from people who found a Pilot Light Lover who was a stranger, a close or casual friend, a friend of the deceased, a lover from the distant past, or someone met on a dating site. There are no rules, no website where Pilot Light Lovers can advertise and find each other. (Come to think of it, that would be a very good idea!)

Acquaintance Sex

Is there someone already in your world who would be willing and able to light your sexual kindling? Someone who has been particularly attentive lately or in the past? Someone who expressed being sexually attracted to you? Depending on the kind of friendship you have and how easily you can express your feelings to this person, you might plan some private time together. It might develop like the following.

A Griever Shares

"I lost my husband to cancer after thirty-two years of marriage. We were each other's first; we met when I was sixteen. He was a sweet, gentle man, a wonderful husband. After he died, I missed having someone I could touch—a gentle sweep of a hand across your partner's back as you walk by, a hug or kiss in the middle of the day for no reason. It took more than two years before I felt like trying to date. The first fellow I had sex with was an old acquaintance. It felt good to be wanted again. The relationship only lasted six months, but it got me back on the horse, so to speak."

A reader commented on my blog,

> "I've been alone for a long time and wonder
> if having sex with someone I'm familiar with
> would be a way for me to feel comfortable
> enough to start dating again. Trying this
> experiment with an old lover might not be a
> good idea, but I feel like using him to get back
> in the game while I try to meet someone I can
> really be with."

Is it "using" someone? Yes, in the strict sense.
But if you're honest about wanting to experience
sex again but not being ready for an ongoing
relationship, your potential sex partner may think
this is a wonderful idea. If not, it won't work with
this person. Have a candid conversation about
what each of you wants and doesn't want, and
make sure you agree.

Just a Hookup

> "I didn't even think about sex for a solid year after
> my husband Dennis died. I spent a lot of time at
> home alone crying. Then two of my dearest friends

got married in a weekend-long celebration. I met a divorced man there and spent the weekend fucking him. I had sex in a hotel with someone I wouldn't ever see again. I had dreaded the wedding because Dennis should have been there celebrating with me, and he wasn't. Having sex for the first time since he died was a great way to distract myself. It was easy for me to pretend that I was someone other than the Widow Who Is Agonizing Over the Absence of Her Husband."

—Heidi Mastrogiovanni, author of *Lala Pettibone's Act Two* and *Lala Pettibone: Standing Room Only*

Maybe you don't want an ongoing relationship—even if temporary. Maybe you just want a break from your sadness and isolation via the feel-good brain chemicals of sexual arousal and release. You want sex with a stranger to get you over the hump, so to speak. And then you want the person to go away. Done.

Be Smart

Enjoy your Pilot Light Lover fully—but don't make the mistake of thinking that because you were able to let go sexually with this new person, this means you're in love again. Your sexual brain and body are firing again, and that's powerful, but that's not the same as love. Be wary of making this relationship more than it is, and don't make any life decisions because of it. Don't move in together, or marry, or open your bank account. Be wary of making any decision that you can't get out of easily if the relationship goes sour, or if one or both of you wants to move on.

Even if this is a transitory affair or a one-time hookup, The Pilot Light Lover's gifts are valuable, and you'll use them as you move forward in your healing:

- The knowledge that you can be sexual with another person and it works;
- The realization that you are desirous and desired;

- The discovery that your body can respond to someone who is not your dead beloved;

- The reminder that sex feels good.

"Whether this new woman would be long-term or not wasn't important; she was kindling new life in him, physically and emotionally, and he was now hopeful in a way he'd never been before. There is an intimacy that only sex can create, where rational thought is suspended and animal instincts take over...."

—Julia Samuel, in *Grief Works: Stories of Life, Death, and Surviving*

Your Takeaway

If you feel ready for a Pilot Light Lover, how do you imagine this happening? Do you want an encounter with a pleasure-giving stranger? A friend? Do you have anyone in mind? Create a "yes," "maybe," and "absolutely not" list of what you do and do not want.

CHAPTER 11

Friends with Benefits

"In 2013, 58 percent of men and 50 percent of women in our 'Singles in America' study reported that they had had a friends-with-benefits relationship, including one in three people in their seventies."

—Helen Fisher, PhD, in *Anatomy of Love: A Natural History of Mating, Marriage, and Why We Stray*, revised edition, 2016

After we lose our mate, most of us will not find ourselves in another love-filled, committed relationship quickly. Does that mean we should deny ourselves partnered sex until Cupid's arrow strikes again? Some of us do choose celibacy until we're in a new love relationship, but many of us prefer to get sexual as soon as we feel physically and emotionally ready for erotic human contact. In some cases, a sexual friend, aka a "friend with benefits" (or FWB), is our solution.

Although some people use "hookup" and "friend with benefits" interchangeably, I see them as quite different. A hookup is a one-time sexual encounter: sex only, no dating, no emotional involvement, and generally no plans for a next time (though that can vary). FWB, however is a sexual connection within a real friendship: a sex buddy. It's more ongoing than a Pilot Light Lover (see Chapter 10), although it may start out as that. We may feel an intimate emotional bond with our FWB, with no expectation or desire that the relationship become more than it is. That's how I experienced my FWB, and I treasure the memory.

A Griever Shares

"I missed male companionship, and about a year after my husband passed, I joined an online dating site. I met several men, but none developed into a sexual relationship. I did, however, deepen a friendship with one of my husband's oldest and dearest friends, and he and I became intimate a few months ago. Experiencing that rush of endorphins again was revitalizing and life-affirming. It seemed so natural and comfortable to extend our friendship in that direction, with shared grieving over someone we had both loved so much."

Five years passed after Robert's death. I kept myself sexually active with my vibrators—even reviewing sex toys "from a senior perspective" on my blog. (I know, a tough job, but somebody's got to do it!) I had tried a few times to get sexual with another human being with varying degrees of success (see Chapter 3, **My Own Struggle with Sex after Grief** and Chapter 7, **It's Okay If You're Not Ready**), but these relationships weren't quite right and didn't continue.

I wasn't looking for love, but I *was* looking for satisfying sex without commitment or expectations for the future. My ideal sex buddy would be an interesting man who pleasured me in bed, held my interest out of bed, and genuinely cared for me as a friend, yet didn't want us to be a couple. He would not demand much of my time, but when we were together, we would be completely focused on each other. Then he would go away until the next time.

In other words, I wanted a "friend with benefits," with as much emphasis on "friend" as on "benefits." Was it realistic to find this, especially at age sixty-nine?

A Griever Shares

"I am sixty-six and lost my husband four months ago, after forty-one years together. I have a very strong sex drive and am at a loss as to how to satisfy it. I do schedule time to have singular sex and find that gratifying. But I miss the intimacy—hugs, kisses, holding hands, with possible lead-up to having oral sex or intercourse. With my sexual energy at a very high level, I wonder if it is too soon to start exploring relationships. I am not ready to commit to someone beyond being 'friends with benefits.' If I'm honest and open about what I want, then it should be up to me, not what societal norms might dictate, to choose when it is appropriate for me. Is four months too soon?"

Lover from the Past

I scoured OkCupid, the dating site where I had met a couple of interesting men. I didn't feel I could say in my profile, "seeking great sex and a decent friendship," because that would bring out the trolls and creeps who salivated at the word "sex" without being my match in any way.

I scrolled through profile after profile, and then my mouse stopped on one of them. I was looking at the photo of a man who had been my lover for nine months about fifteen years earlier. The relationship had ended without animosity, and we had taken walks together occasionally to catch up since then. In his candid profile, he described being in a committed, ethically nonmonogamous relationship. His agreement with his partner allowed him to have a sexual friendship with someone else, but only if it was no threat to the primary relationship. He was looking for a FWB.

Perfect. Here was someone I already knew, liked, and trusted. He understood—and liked—that I was ready for a friendship that included sex and affection, but not one that had the goal of developing into something more. That fit exactly what he needed, too, though for different reasons. We made a date to walk and talk, explored a long kiss, and made a date to meet again—in my bedroom. This began a sweet, sexy, and friendly affair that continued for more than two years.

From Joan's Grief Journal, August 2013:

> *"The sweet combination of new and familiar.*
> *I can finally move forward and touch another*
> *person's skin with pleasure and without*
> *comparison or sadness. I feel like I've emerged*
> *from a very long time in a cocoon."*

How We Made It Work

A friends-with-benefits relationship needs more than just an agreement to have sex without strings. For us, these steps and agreements made it work.

1. **Honesty.** We were honest with ourselves and with each other about what the relationship was and was not. He was also honest with his primary partner.

2. **Clear communication.** Each encounter started with talking and ended with talking, with sex in the middle. (A sex sandwich?)

3. **Sexual generosity.** We were each intent on giving pleasure as much as receiving it.

4. **Safer Sex.** We agreed on condoms and dental dams (see Chapter 8, Your (New) First Time) right from the beginning, and we never wavered.

5. **Laughter.** We laughed when he shared a fantasy about a sexual position, only to have me tell him my old knees wouldn't allow it. We laughed when seeing the film *50 Shades of Grey* together got us *out* of the mood for sex. Things that might have

been setbacks were reasons for giggles and compassion instead.

6. **Interest in each other.** His profession and mine led to sharing interesting stories. Enjoying how the other's brain worked intensified the sexual delight.

More about number 1, honesty: Long before we pulled down the bed covers, we discussed our expectations and agreements about the relationship and its ramifications. For example, his partner had veto power—if at any point she was uncomfortable with our relationship, or a date that we had scheduled conflicted with something she wanted to do with him, he would cancel with me. I was free to pursue any interest in other men, date, and have sex with others.

You may ask what the point is of having a sex buddy if you continue to date others and potentially become sexual with them. The point is to enjoy sex, to nurture that part of ourselves, and not to let sexual hunger make us jump into wrong relationships!

Our FWB arrangement lasted about two years. We changed our relationship back to platonic friends when we agreed our sexual relationship had fulfilled what we each needed and it was time to move on. He had met someone on whom he wanted to focus without distraction, and I was ready to open myself to meeting new men. I could do that while I was with him—there was no exclusivity in our agreement. But ironically, I felt that having this relationship that sexually satisfied me left me less interested in taking the time and effort to find and date new people, which I knew needed to be my direction next.

I am grateful to this man who was my dear friend with benefits.

Your Takeaway

Would a friend with benefits work for you? List the pros and cons of this kind of relationship for you personally. How would you communicate this to a potential lover?

CHAPTER 12

After Caregiving Your Partner

"[I]f you have been that caregiver who was looking after an ill spouse with a fatal diagnosis, you may have started grieving long before he died. To people on the outside of your personal experience—even your children—it may look like it is too soon after your husband's death to start a relationship. However, if you have been caring for him and watching him fade away, you may be quite ready to move on into other relationships."

—Kristen Meekhof and James Windell,
in *A Widow's Guide to Healing: Gentle Support and Advice for the First 5 Years*

Although the book quoted above was written specifically for widows, the message is not restricted to one gender. Mourning can start long before death when a partner has an incurable illness. When sex ends long before death, this loss, added to the physical and emotional toll that caregiving takes, can be excruciating. After death—or sometimes before death—sex may happen quickly for the surviving partner.

The caregiver may seem to others to be moving on too quickly, not grieving long enough or correctly. Please know that you're not grieving wrong if you're ready to reach out for the comfort of sex and the uplift of a new relationship. You've been grieving for a long time already. If you don't feel ready, though, honor that self-knowledge and wait until it's time.

In other words, don't impose anyone else's rules on your own timeline.

A Griever Shares

"My grief started a long time before my spouse died. He had leukemia for fourteen years, then dementia kicked in. After he passed away, I resurrected my libido with a vibrator, cannabis, and Joan Price's books. My sexual awakening was redirected to a former boyfriend who came back into my life. I am almost seventy-three and vibrant. I have wisdom and experience. I am having the life I always dreamed of."

Moving Back toward Sex and Pleasure

A perspective from Cyndi Darnell, clinical sexologist and relationship therapist

After death, we may feel relieved that our loved one's suffering is over, especially if the death was protracted and complicated. We may experience a sense of coming back into ourselves after a hiatus from being a caregiver.

For many people caring for an infirm lover, grief begins well before death. When death comes, we may feel a release for ourselves as well as for our loved one. This may make us feel guilty because we feel we *should* be sad, and we think we are not sad enough. We are not *showing* enough loss.

Our culture has few grieving and death rituals, but many social expectations. How long before we move on? How much grief should we display? Navigating our own bodies, needs, and desires becomes even further complicated. Shame often compounds grief. We may feel guilty for wanting sex with another, or even for wanting sex at all, as if that would dilute the relationship with our beloved who has passed. Such emotions may block our willingness or ability to move toward exploration.

When moving back toward sex and pleasure, use the body as the tool for deciding what is going to feel best, tuning into your "felt sense." Is pleasure what I long for right now? Is it sexual pleasure I seek? If the answer is yes, then start by bringing sex back as solo practice.

Sometimes peak sexual experiences can trigger floods of tears, tenderness, and vulnerability. Don't be alarmed, but do pay attention to what your body is telling you. You may want to reach out to a therapist or coach for support during an experience like this.

"Anticipatory Sexual Bereavement": Grieving When Your Partner Is Still Alive

"When a loved one dies after a lengthy illness, those around her might experience something called 'anticipatory grief.' It suggests that at least some of your grieving might be done in advance of the passing of this person...Widows and widowers who have endured a long struggle cannot wait to reengage with life once again. Their reentry into work and social life can be a little shocking to those around them as they expect a long intensive grieving period to follow."

—Fred Colby, in *Widower to Widower: Surviving the End of Your Most Important Relationship*

Grief starts long before a beloved dies when a long, chronic illness or untreatable, progressive condition thrusts the healthy partner into the role of caregiver.

Sex becomes impossible, either due to the illness or because of the shift from lover or spouse to a patient/caregiver relationship. Caregivers may experience "anticipatory sexual bereavement" and start grieving for lost intimacy and sexual connection while the ill partner still lives. Caregivers often feel guilty about these feelings.

A Griever Shares

"My 'anticipatory sexual bereavement' began to surface during my wife's long illness, about three years before she died. The only person I could share this with was my sister, who was my confidante. I was able to air my horniness, frustration, sadness, and ache-for-my-beloved with someone I trusted. I could say to her, 'I love sex, I miss sex, and I'm so damned horny

I could spit.' I didn't do anything about my frustration beyond solo sex, but it was good to have someone to listen nonjudgmentally and understand."

When I conceived this book, I thought it would be exclusively for and about people whose partners have died, because there's no book out there that deals specifically with sex after the death of a beloved. However, I expanded my topic when I heard from grievers whose partners still live but are so ill or physically compromised that the relationship is only about caregiving these days.

For decades, I've known people in this situation. Their daily lives and emotional lives are devoted to taking care of their partners. But what about the caregivers' needs? Caregivers are often told that they can only care for their partners if they care for themselves, too. They're encouraged to take breaks for solitude, friends, activities, and exercise. But what about sex? What about joining with another human being who can give and receive pleasure and bond with you in joy? What about the relief and respite that sex can bring?

A Griever Shares

"My partner was ill for two years before he died of AIDS in 1992. We had an open arrangement because of his illness, so I was already sexual with other men. I remember using sex as a way to deal with some of the grief, connecting with a sex friend about a week after my partner died. Maybe it was my way to recreate a human connection."

Often spousal/partner caregivers who seek out the balance of a new relationship do so in secret because their families, friends, and religious communities would shame them if they knew. I wish we lived in a society that was less judgmental and less hypocritical. I hope that by sharing these candid stories, we can start to change this cultural attitude.

A Griever Shares

"My husband is still alive, but he has dementia. I am his primary caregiver and his advocate, and I love him greatly in a complicated way. This is anticipatory grieving in all its glory. Some months ago, I entered the world of online dating. I was lucky enough to meet a man with whom I have fallen in love, and it's reciprocal. He, too, is a caregiver for his longtime partner, who has cancer. We understand each other's constraints without having to negotiate them, since they are nonnegotiable. We are very lucky to have found each other, although our lives are both hot messes."

Support Groups

A caregivers' support group can be very helpful. These people understand what you're going through—often better than your most loving friends and family. Some group leaders welcome discussions about sex—others do not. A support group is not intended to be used as a dating mixer, but some people have told me that friendships with benefits started there. Whether that happens for you or not, just being able to share what you're going through can be helpful.

Other people, though, have described support groups in which sex was the elephant in the room. This is true for grief support groups as well as caregivers' groups. One man told me that he announced to his group, "I'm so horny!" He said that some were shocked, others laughed, and one woman gave him a long, meaningful look. (Sorry, he didn't share what happened after that.)

A Griever Shares

"I wish there were a network of spousal caregivers of a 'certain age' for exploring the possibility of sexual relationships with other caregivers: a dating service for spousal caregivers, so to speak. I'm a seventy-year-old longtime caregiver for my wife, who is physically disabled and cognitively impaired. I love her and intend to take care of her as long as I can, but our relationship ceased to be sexual about fifteen years ago. I've had a couple of long-term relationships with other women during my caregiver journey. The last one ended more than two years ago, and I have not had sex since then, other than solo. I'm a longtime member of a support group for spousal caregivers. Lack of intimacy in our lives is unacknowledged. If there were only some way to find other spousal caregivers who seek intimate relationships outside of their marriages!"

An Unusual Solution

Current and former spousal caregivers usually tell me about either their horniness or their lack of interest in sex when the ill partner is no longer able to be sexual. Both reactions are valid, and I hope you can accept and honor your feelings without judgment. This story was unusual in that this couple found a creative way to keep their sexual intimacy:

A Griever Shares

"My wife passed from ovarian cancer after surviving for two years. When she was too sick for any sexual activity, I was more concerned about how she felt, and sex was not on my mind. If I got horny, I masturbated. We developed a system. If she found herself sexually stimulated, she turned on a special light as a signal. Then she verbalized what she wanted me to do. I was glad to please her. Sometimes she talked me through masturbation, sometimes it was oral stimulation. When she was in remission, it was anything goes. Experimentation was high on her list, and I was happy to see her smile and enjoy herself. What brought me the most joy was knowing that I was not being selfish and that the time I had left with her was hers."

Your Takeaway

Don't judge yourself if you have strong sexual feelings during and/or soon after caregiving your beloved. This is natural and healthy. Find a nonjudgmental confidant or counselor with whom you can discuss your feelings. Remember—your timeline is your own. No one else decides when you're ready to bring sex back into your life.

CHAPTER 13

Massage or More?

"Seeing a sex worker is more than just sex. Sometimes it's about getting some of the feel-good brain chemicals back. Touch involves the hormone oxytocin, and sex is a complex mix of oxytocin, dopamine, and vasopressin. In my experience, seeing a sex worker during grief brings out a level of vulnerability. By making a booking, you are cementing the decision to recognize your need to be open, to feel. If you are unsure about seeing a sex worker when you are grieving, wait. We can't fix things for you or make things right. But when you are ready, we can help you to feel connected to a human again, with no judgment or expectations."

—Corrine, www.thelovelycorrine.com, Tasmania, Australia

My Erotic Massage

On my sixty-sixth birthday, after a year and a half of celibacy (other than my sex toys), I bought myself an erotic massage. It was the best gift ever. I wasn't ready for reciprocal sex with a partner, and I wasn't ready for intercourse. But I was ready for the physical and emotional bouquet of pleasures that I received from this massage:

- The sweet, unhurried touch of a pleasure-giving man

- The surprise of feeling my life force emerge and bloom

- The amazement that my body was still capable of shivering and screaming joy

- The relief of sexual release

I wrote about this experience in *Naked at Our Age*, and I expanded on the sexy details when it was selected for *Best Sex Writing 2012*. I heard from many people who wanted to know how to get this experience for themselves, and from others who chided me not for only doing it but for writing about it. A widower on a first date—who happened to have read *Naked at Our Age*—said he thought what I did was wrong. That first date was a last date. *Tip*: If someone judges you, drop them immediately. Their judgment has nothing to do with you and everything to do with them. (See Chapter 2, **Myths about Sex and Grieving**, for more.)

A Griever Shares

"My wife's illness ended our once active sex life two years before her death. I masturbated and watched porn, but I became extremely lonesome for a woman's caresses and the feel of a woman's body next to mine. I had no idea how to meet the kind of age-appropriate women I might like to date. I considered hiring a sex worker to satisfy my need. But when I searched online for escort services and sex workers in my area, I found photographs of attractive, alluring women, but all of them were much younger than my seventy plus years. Horny as I was, sex for hire with someone less than half my age didn't feel right, so

I didn't take the step. Then I discovered the www.
maturesensual.sexy directory. They weren't my
age, but at least many were over forty-five."

Hiring a Professional

When you think about hiring the services of a sex
worker or a massage therapist who is willing to
provide the touch you crave and a happy ending,
does it entice you? Our sex-negative society makes
it difficult (and, depending on the services being
offered, often illegal) for professionals to advertise
that they provide services with a sexual release
outcome. You may need to read between the lines.

Figure out exactly what you'd like to experience
and what search terms you might use to find
the right professional. For example, to find a
massage where genitals are not off limits, you
might Google one of these terms plus your city or
state: erotic massage, sensual massage, full-body
sensual massage, Tantric massage, yoni massage
(for vulva), lingam massage (for penis).

A Griever Shares

"When I booked a full-body, sensual Tantra massage with a woman who advertised online, I wasn't sure what to expect. She made it clear in advance that sexual intercourse was not in the cards. That was fine with me. I was eager to experience an erotic massage and curious to learn more about Tantra, so I agreed to pay her significant fee for the adventure. I was not disappointed! The interactions throughout were lovely and erotic, the massage itself was memorable, and my orgasm—produced by her manual stimulation of my genitals—was extremely satisfying. After my wife's death, this erotic massage helped me see myself as once again a fully functioning sexual being."

Is a Surrogate Partner for You?

A surrogate partner is a trained professional who works therapeutically with clients who need help with physical and emotional intimacy, including interacting sexually. Surrogate partners usually work with clients via referrals from therapists, creating a three-person team to work on sexual and intimacy issues. If you're interested and you don't have a therapist who will refer you, Google "surrogate partner" plus your city or state, or consult a surrogate directory, such as www.surrogatetherapy.org and others serving local regions. Some surrogate partners work independently and advertise on their own websites.

A Griever Shares

"After my wife, the true love of my life, died, I felt so alone—crying, screaming, shrieking about this hole in my heart. There was a sexual component to my grief. But where could I go, what could I do? I overcame my inhibitions and contacted a surrogate partner. This turned out to be one of the best decisions of my life. At our first meeting, I poured out personal sexual information like a spy on truth serum. Sometimes we need a special someone with whom we can feel safe who has no agenda except to help us. Intimate time with a surrogate goes hand in hand with talk. Skin on skin contact is therapeutic. Being naked and breast to breast, holding each other as tight as you can, frees up so much emotion. This intimate time is nothing like casual sex. Your surrogate, by definition, is a replacement partner for a mutually agreed time period. The purpose is to help you move forward with your life."

Can a Surrogate Partner Help You?

A perspective from Kendra Holliday, surrogate partner in St Louis, MO, www.beopenandhonest.com

As a surrogate partner, one of my roles is to help people who are in transition heal and move forward with their lives. Sometimes they are in transition because they have lost a loved one. The way they lost their loved one can make a difference in their grieving process. Those who lost someone suddenly can take longer to recover, whereas those who assumed a caregiver role in the last few months or years of their partner's lives tend to be ready sooner to seek new intimate experiences. They had time during the caregiving period to process their grief and think about what they want going forward.

The biggest challenge I see is survivor guilt. They feel guilty about having another chance at intimate relationships, and they worry about replacing their loved one. That is why so many people choose to remain celibate. I like teaching them that they are not *replacing love,* they are *adding to love.*

Many avoid dating because they don't want to get married again, which is society's expectation. I teach them to think about what they want in their new relationships. They don't need to fall into old patterns. They can design their own relationship, on their own terms.

In the process of self-discovery, it's good to address skin hunger, whether through massage therapy, surrogate partner work, a cuddle companion, or a friend with benefits. I help them brush up on their intimacy skills, learn new techniques, and address issues they may be having. They gain confidence as they prepare themselves for the next chapter in their lives.

Your Takeaway

Would it help you to hire a professional who understands that you're grieving and craving touch? Figure out what form you want that touch to take. Explore the possibilities in your area.

CHAPTER 14

Sex of Many Stripes

"Grieving people often try to connect to their erotic side in an effort to push back the feeling of deadness. Our sex drive is the playful, creative part of ourselves that seeks out vitality and unpredictability. It may also be a source of comfort for people who have been left feeling alone and cut off from others; it is very common for people to want to hold someone close when the fragility of their world threatens to overwhelm them."

—Julia Samuel, in *Grief Works: Stories of Life, Death, and Surviving*

Although I've organized this book thematically, many grievers sent me experiences and beliefs that don't fit in neat boxes—or into neat chapter titles. Grievers wrote me about casual encounters, sexual adventures, previous agreements with their deceased partners, struggles with what's allowed and what isn't, and personal ways of defining relationships. These all fit under the "no one way is the right way" and "everyone grieves differently and reenters sex differently" themes of this book, but otherwise might seem to have little in common.

If you have read this far and come away with, "but that's not me exactly," I invite you to explore what you personally want and need at this point in your grieving process and at this stage of your life. You may need a temporary solution, or you may be ready to make a big change in the kind of sexual experience you're ready to explore.

Read these grievers' experiences with an open mind. Some may seem far from your personal sex life, desires, or beliefs, and others may attract or resonate with you.

A Griever Shares

"My husband passed away when I was fifty. We had been together since I was fourteen, and he was my only partner. After some months, I just went for it. Looking back now, perhaps I acted too quickly, but I felt like a teenager again, but with more experience and no worry about getting pregnant. My partners were all very different experiences, body shapes, and sizes. My current partner has very interesting sexual habits, which I like, and some of them are new to me. My sex life is now fantastic—though in a different way from my lovely intimacy with my much-loved husband."

Hookup Sex

"Across our SIA [Singles in America 2013] studies, men and women in their sixties had engaged in just as many fleeting encounters as those in their twenties and thirties."

—Helen Fisher, PhD, in *Anatomy of Love: A Natural History of Mating, Marriage, and Why We Stray*

If you're feeling drawn to no-strings sex with strangers because it pulls you out of your grief for an hour—or because you just enjoy sex that way—please don't seek advice from the judgmental, self-proclaimed grief experts online or in books, articles, and blogs. You'll likely encounter what one griever called "opinionated bullshit" which attempts to shame you for wanting sex without a relationship. The Internet is an enormous resource for good information and helpful advice, but it's also a source of misinformation and horrid advice which I hope you avoid. As I've repeated throughout this book, no one but you can decide when it's time to recharge your sex life, or with whom, or what kind of sex that should be.

We're often seen as being a minute away from making awful decisions because...well... people in grief often *do* make bad decisions. Our brains are not running on all cylinders. That's why we're advised not to decide anything big or irreversible while we're in grief. But does hookup sex have to be a major decision requiring input from others? No, or maybe, depending on your views about sex. It's really no one's business but yours if that's the direction that makes you feel better.

You need to be smart about it: safe sex always, choose someone who's kind and sexually giving, let a trusted friend know where you are and with whom—you know the drill, and you're fully capable of determining and going after the kind of sex you want.

A Griever Shares

"As for what ended my celibacy, I was just ready. I had married very young, having had no chance to explore my sexuality. After my husband died, I took to wild sex like a duck to water. I had sex with dozens of men in the first two years, many a one-time thing at a party. I was a kid in a candy store. In the past twelve years, I've been with maybe sixty men or more."

When casual encounters are your choice, I see nothing wrong with that. But some grievers wrote me in frustration because they found hookup sex, but they were really looking for a more intimate connection.

A Griever Shares

"I'm seventy-four and sexually active. My wife of thirty-four years passed away fourteen years ago. I decided that I didn't want to spend the rest of my life alone. I needed to find the last love of my life, and the rest would flow from there. For a time, I was 'on tour.' I met a lot of women and had sex with them, but there was always something missing—the spark that I wanted in my relationship. I wanted to be head-over-heels in love again, and it didn't happen. I found that although I was sincerely looking for a committed relationship, it was a lot easier to find sex than it was to find love on the Internet."

Exploring Your Kinks

A Griever Shares

"I have been asked to participate in sexual adventures by several dominant escorts. I did enjoy them. While feeling ashamed, I was excited at the same time, and I loved listening to a powerful female's voice telling me what to do."

Sex advice columnist and podcaster Dan Savage often divides people who enjoy kink (unconventional, offbeat, or edgy sexual practices) into two categories:

- Those who always knew they were kinky.

- Those who explored kink because they wanted to be GGG (good, giving, and game) with a kinky partner—and discovered they liked it.

Some grievers report that they had conventional (aka "vanilla") sex with their longtime partner, and now they're learning that they find

kinky sexual experiences the most exciting
and satisfying:

Poly, Submissive, and Grieving

*A perspective from Jade Melisande, sex, kink, and
relationship blogger at www.piecesofjade.blog*

I was in a poly, dominant/submissive (D/s)
relationship with W for seven years before
he died. Kink was such an integral part of
my relationship with W that when he died, I
felt like part of me had died with him. I had
identified not just as *a* submissive, but as *his*
submissive. I didn't know what I-without-

him looked like in the world in general, and especially in the kink world. How could I be a submissive when my dominant was gone? W and I had a connection that I knew I could never find with anyone else. That's a whole lot to ask anyone else to deal with. Did I even want to try?

My steps back into kink and recovering my sexuality were slow and timid. I knew what I liked. I knew what I wanted. I knew that it would take someone special to capture and hold my interest—if we could even get past the big gaping wounds that losing W had left in me.

Eventually, I did connect with someone who drew me out of myself enough to play again, kink-wise and sexually. Surprising us both, we ended up in a deep D/s relationship, not just play partners. We've been together four years now.

Open Relationship with Rules

Sex after death of a beloved is sometimes a continuation of an open-relationship agreement made while the partner was alive. Maybe the relationship was always nonexclusive, or maybe that agreement happened after one person became ill. The couple talked honestly about the sexual needs of the healthy partner and made an agreement, with whatever restrictions felt right to them: sexual interaction only with others, no emotional connection? Only with friends? Only one-time hookups? Don't ask, don't tell? Tell me every detail? Have sex as a threesome? As in every kind of sexual agreement, people make their own rules.

After the partner dies, sometimes the griever wants to maintain the agreement and keep sex with others separate from the kind of intimacy shared with the beloved, at least for now.

Sex with Restrictions: A Griever Shares

My husband was a longtime AIDS survivor. We were together twenty years and married when gay marriage became legal in California in 2008. His terminal illness and medications affected his ability to have sex, often preventing him from getting or maintaining an erection. We had an open sex life, with my husband's encouragement. Sometimes I would have sex with someone we both knew who was comfortable having my husband present, in this way including him, if only visually.

After my husband's passing, it took about a year before I became sexually active again. I never felt guilt but was often sad. I missed the intimacy: caressing the back of his neck, holding hands, hand on knee, long embraces. I still reach for him in bed, longing to feel him near.

I'm sexually active now, but I do have some restrictions. My sex partners are men who are in an open, committed relationship, usually married. This way the relationship cannot become more than sexual. I won't allow anyone to sleep overnight. I did that once and couldn't sleep. The body next to me wasn't my husband, and it felt wrong. It took more than two years before I could take a shower with another man, an intimacy I only shared with my husband. I won't share one sexual position that was my husband's favorite.

When an open relationship starts before death, the survivor may find it easy to get back to partnered sex, but may still be lonely for an intimate connection:

Mourning Loss of Intimacy: A Griever Shares

I'm a former priest. I married the love of my life. My husband died a year ago, and I'll always be grateful for the love that he brought me. He was very sexual with a high libido and was hot and passionate in our lovemaking. Then out of the blue, as if a switch had been turned off in him, he had no sex drive whatsoever. This was due to his illness, but we didn't know that. While we tried to figure it out, our marriage became celibate. After about three months of no sex, he told me that it was okay for me to have sex with other men. His only caveat was that I tell him beforehand, and then, afterwards, he wanted to know all the details.

Soon after he made our marriage an open marriage, he began to get sick and I had no opportunity nor desire to be with another man sexually. Following his death, sex with another man was the last thing on my mind.

It was several months after he died that I began to reawaken my interest in sexual intimacy with another man. I began to have one-night-stand encounters. The sex satiated my carnal desire but was not making love. There was no intimacy or deep connection. My sexual desire has since waned significantly, but I still yearn to have an intimate connection with another man, if only to hold, kiss and snuggle.

You may have noticed that two griever stories in this section happen to be from gay men, but neither your gender nor your orientation defines the kind of agreement you and your partner make.

When It Was Bad Before

Most of the grievers who contributed to this book were in love with their deceased partners and miss them powerfully. But some were in relationships that were abusive, destructive or just sexually unfulfilling. Their partner's death was a release in part, though the feelings were usually complicated. Here are some of their experiences:

Grievers Share

"I think I always knew there was something missing sexually during my marriage. We weren't open to much experimentation, then my husband had his first heart attack at thirty-one. I was five months pregnant. Keeping him alive and employed seemed much more important than exploring sexual fantasies. Looking back, we were not big on communication in bed. I'm not sure that I was aware that I longed for something more. I certainly wasn't aware of what it was."

*

"I was forty-five when my husband of twenty-three years passed away from a terminal illness. Our marriage was so fraught with gaslighting, brainwashing, and emotional abuse that I don't know how I survived. The relief of no longer being emotionally abused gave me peace to begin dating, which has been liberating for me. I've been in a new relationship for two and a half years. I didn't expect the flashbacks of repressed sexual abuse. My boyfriend holds me and lets me cry while I process what happened. Sometimes I let him know that I'm dealing with grief and emotions and I'll talk about them when I'm ready. Those instances don't happen as often as they did when we began dating."

"My husband passed away two years ago. Sex had not been very good in the marriage. I lived in a very conservative area where the men were boss, they made the decisions, their needs always came first. The last nine years, there was no sex in my marriage. I was raised in an era when 'nice girls didn't talk about sex.' How was a girl supposed to be a virgin on her wedding day and totally hot, accomplished, and eager on her wedding night? I have never figured that out."

*

"My husband of forty-eight years died after fifteen years of Alzheimer's. It was not a wonderful marriage, and I never had an orgasm with him. If I ever tried to take the lead in sex, this scared him and completely turned him off. I learned to stuff it and was angry. My orgasms were alone with a vibrator. About four months after my husband died, I was driving, and the newscaster said, 'It turns out that January is the most popular month for people to join dating apps.' I promptly joined a few, and at age seventy-four, I am engaged to a wonderful guy. What an amazing time we have! My advice to others—go for it! Don't wait!"

Your Takeaway

What do *you* personally need at this time? Divide a page into three columns:

- "I know I want...."

- "I might want to explore...."

- "I know I don't want...."

Don't censor—just write what comes out. See what you learn about yourself.

Journaling Your Journey

"In those early days, writing was how I connected with Matt, how I continued our conversation that was so abruptly stopped. It was how I recorded rare moments of calm, of feeling loved and grounded, places I could go back to and relive when everything had gone too dark to be endured. It was where I recorded those dark moments, too. On the page, everything is allowed. Everything has a voice."

—Megan Devine, in *It's OK that You're Not OK: Meeting Grief and Loss in a Culture that Doesn't Understand*

Two months after Robert died, I decided to keep a journal. I had journaled my way through hard times in my life in the past, and it was time to use this tool again. But I was immobilized every time I started because I was torn between two needs that seemed to conflict:

keeping the good memories of Robert alive and chronicling the awfulness of the grief that enveloped me.

Solution: I decided to keep two separate journals—a Memory Journal and a Grief Journal. I would write in one, then put it down, grab the other, and write in that one. Some days I wrote only memories, other days I wrote only grief, but usually I wrote both. I often wrote *to* Robert, as if I were talking to him.

Keeping the journals separate was perfect for me, and I heartily recommend it to you. Here's why:

- The memories of my beloved were pristine and untainted by the bad stuff.

- I could read the Memory Journal anytime I wanted to relive the good times.

- Sometimes when I sat down to write in the Memory Journal, I was convinced that I had recorded all the memories already and there was nothing more to write. Then a new one would come to me, and I was comforted to know that I would never run out of memories.

- I found over the next two years that the Memory Journal contained moments that I would have forgotten had I not recorded them. I loved reading it.
I still do.

- The Grief Journal was a place to express my raw, soul-searing, wailing grief.

- Writing in my Grief Journal calmed me down at times I felt out of control.

- By writing in my Grief Journal when I felt horrible and when I felt a little better, I discovered the activities that helped me lighten my grief: exercise, walking with close friends, dancing, small accomplishments, and, yes, writing in both journals.

- I made notes in my Grief Journal after appointments with my grief counselors so that I could think about their advice and put it into action.

- By recording in my Grief Journal my thoughts about and steps toward dating and intimacy again, I now have a chronicle of how that happened for me: the fits and starts and retreats and trying again. That became the foundation for this book: sharing what I learned.

For the first three years, I wrote regularly. At first, it was daily, or almost that often. I would write in one journal, switch to the other, and cry as I wrote. Later, I wrote less often, but it was still a regular habit. When my sadness overwhelmed me, or when I felt I was standing at the edge of a cliff wondering whether to jump, I wrote. As my life normalized (the "new normal," in grief parlance), I would jot notes every so often, maybe weekly, then monthly, and later, maybe once or twice a year, just to record how I was doing, or else to give myself a safe place to be raw and real, like this entry:

From Joan's Grief Journal:

*"4/13/2011. Today I cry alone in my bathrobe.
Sometimes it feels like other people have
forgotten you, or think you've moved beyond
your grief, or that you should. But I haven't.
I'm functioning in public, not always in
private. Often, I say honestly, 'I love my life.'
But at times, like today, I'm lost and sad, crying
and calling out to you. 'Come back,' I plead.
'Don't be dead anymore!'"*

Even though I write for a living, using a computer
and all the tech tools available to me, I write my
journals in longhand: old-style pen on paper.
Somehow writing this slower way elicits thoughts
that come from the heart more than from the
brain. I rediscover memories I had forgotten. I
access deeper feelings.

Now, a decade after Robert's death, I rarely feel
the need to write in my journals, but I do love
reading the Memory Journal. The Grief Journal
accomplished what it was supposed to for me,
and I was finally able to put it away. Returning to

it to make notes for this book, I went into a tear-filled, dark place rereading it. But this time, it was a dark place with a light switch. And I knew how to find my path out into the sunshine.

"In grief...many widows return to their diary to give voice to pent-up, unspoken feelings at a time when their emotions and thoughts are unclear and acutely private. What is whirling around in one's head now is too new and immediate and too confusing for voicing. Keeping a diary—or journal, as they are now more often called—can be a lifesaver."

—Genevieve Davis Ginsburg, in *Widow to Widow: Thoughtful, Practical Ideas for Rebuilding Your Life*

10 Tips for Starting Your Memory and Grief Journals

1. Visit your local bookstore and buy yourself two blank journals that appeal to you. Maybe they're especially lovely, or

maybe the cover designs or colors have special meaning.

2.   Decide which one will be your Memory Journal and which one will be your Grief Journal. Name them. Write a few sentences of introduction that describe your purpose.

3.   Create a ritual to set the mood when you write. When I first started, I lit a candle each time.

4.   Date every entry, especially in your Grief Journal. This will be helpful later when you reread your journal and see how far you've come.

5.   Write for as long as you want each time. It might be five minutes; it might be half an hour. Whatever you need is fine.

6.   Don't stop to correct yourself or figure out the best way to say what you feel. Just let it out.

7. When you don't think you have anything
   to say, reread some earlier entries
   for inspiration.

8. Don't worry if you find yourself repeating
   thoughts you've already written—this is all
   part of the process.

9. Don't censor yourself. Nothing is off limits.

10. Enjoy the process. I know it may seem
    impossible to enjoy recording your grief, but
    strangely, recording it may give you a place
    to put it where it doesn't dominate your
    every moment.

Most of what I wrote my Grief Journal had
nothing to do with reclaiming my sexuality, but
some of it did. It's revealing for me to reread my
entries about sex, because now I can see how this
very slow process worked for me. Here are some
entries specifically about sex and grief:

From Joan's Grief Journal

Nov. 2008: "*Considering getting together with my Magic Wand for the first time since before Robert died three months ago. I hadn't felt the need or the desire before now.*"

Dec. 2008: "*I miss cuddling and the feel and smell of a man more than I miss sex. I can't ever snuggle with Robert or inhale his scent again, and that loss is overwhelming. Missing sex for its own sake isn't strong, but missing sex with Robert because of the total way we melted into each other is soul-searingly powerful.*"

Feb. 2009: "*[A close male friend] and I sat on his couch talking and kissing. I felt marvelous stirrings—marvelous because it felt like I was coming back to life. His kisses, his face, his hand touching mine were his own, not Robert's. I didn't feel (as I had worried) that I was pretending Robert was with me. The experience was totally different, totally separate, and really nice. We didn't go beyond kisses, didn't want to, didn't need to. It was lovely just as it was.*

He told me the "life force" was starting to shine in me again, and this was very attractive and appealing." (*Learn more in the "Fritz" section of Chapter 3,* **My Own Struggle with Sex After Grief.**)

Aug. 2009 [one-year death anniversary]: "I became a sex toy reviewer—such fun. I started really enjoying solo sex. Hey, I can have a sex life on my own! I feel energetic, even sexy, thanks to my buzzing toys and the knowledge that my skin and my life can give me pleasure."

Sept. 2009: "I spent a weekend going to a singles party one night and a date the next. I thought I was ready to dip my toes into dating. I wasn't. It was all wrong. I couldn't wait to be home alone. I have no emotional space available to open to strangers. I don't know when I'll be ready to reenter the world fully."

Nov. 2009: "I'm getting an erotic massage on my birthday! I hope I can get into the spirit of it without crying (much). I've never done anything like this." (See Chapter 13, **Massage or More?***)*

Jan. 2010: "My New Year's Resolutions include getting social and meeting new men—not because I want to (or even think I could) fall in love again, but because I do want to be sexual again and feed that part of my mental and physical health."

Aug. 2010: "I had a dream that I announced to all my friends, 'I'm ready to date again.' Am I? What would that be like? Will I recognize the sparkle of an eye, the bounce in a step, the quiet of a listening mind, the joy in a teasing voice, when it's the moment to let a man into my life again? Will sex with someone else be a renewal or a sad reminder?"

Oct. 2010: "I told a friend today that I need to start dating or I'll stay in grief. I need to divert my emotions and bring men into my life. I feel the desire to touch, smell, hear, see, and taste maleness."

Nov. 2010: "I love getting out and doing new things, meeting new people, including men I'm meeting from Match and OkCupid. I've met two *in person, and though neither is likely to lead to intimacy, it's good to connect and learn someone else's story. Sex? Far off, I'm sure. But somewhere in the future."*

Feb. 2011: "Dream: I was finally ready to have sex with a new man. I brought him home but hadn't prepared by straightening my messy house. I asked him to wait in the living room for a minute and I dashed to straighten, but the clutter kept increasing everywhere I looked. It was an impossible task, and my sexual energy completely dissipated, replaced by anxiety. The only spot that was ready was a neat little rectangular basket of condoms, arranged like tea packets in a café. So funny and obvious! My house = my psyche is a mess about bringing someone home."

Oct. 2011: "I need to truly open my heart and my arms to a new man's touch, laughter, smell, and connection—because I want and need that for my own wholeness. It's for me, because it's time."

I strongly recommend journaling your process. Don't rule it out because you're not a professional writer or you've never enjoyed writing. Your emotions, not your intellect, will dictate the words. No one else will read what you write, unless you choose to share it.

A Griever Shares

"Journaling can be extremely therapeutic. Being able to pour out all the anger, guilt, and other negative feelings without being judged is healing. What I've learned through journaling is that pain has to be expressed somehow before we can move forward."

Your Takeaway

Whether or not writing is a comfortable way to express yourself, try the ideas here for starting a Grief Journal and a Memory Journal, separately or together. Don't make it a task—let it be a welcoming place to express yourself.

CHAPTER 16

Grief Counselors, Sex Coaches, and Support Groups

"You are going to hurt! Maybe more than you ever have before... Please hear me on this one thing: Talk to someone. The sooner the better. Don't be a macho fool. Learn to let it out in controlled and constructive ways that will help you to heal... Counseling is critical because there are things that you just don't feel comfortable talking about with your kids, relatives, or friends. If you choose to not talk to anyone about these things, you may delay the grieving process and risk even more severe issues in the future...My counselor provided me with tips on how to deal with some of the issues I was facing and with some assurance that what I was going through was normal and I was not going crazy."

—Fred Colby, in *Widower to Widower: Surviving the End of Your Most Important Relationship*

I would not be the person I am today without the compassion, guidance, wisdom, and shepherding of my grief counselors. I would not have arrived at this place of joy, goals, accomplishment, and ability to give and receive love again without the four people who guided me when I was a sobbing, quivering mess of tears. I owe them much.

During the worst of my grieving, I felt like I was out-of-control crazy, with my brain chemicals going haywire. I felt physically ill as well. In fact, I ended up in the hospital one day with what I thought was a heart attack, so vicious was the searing pain. It turned out to be a broken heart metaphorically, but not physiologically. (But don't ignore this or other symptoms—grievers do get ill.)

This chapter is less about sex and more about getting through grief to be ready for life moving forward, which hopefully will include sex. If you're white-knuckling through your grief, or you've shut down emotionally, or you're numbing yourself with alcohol or drugs, realize that these efforts will not get you past your grief. You'll only delay your healing. Make your own choices, of course, but please read this chapter and think about your options before reacting with, "I don't need counseling."

> "I have regularly seen that it is not the pain of grief that damages individuals...but the things they do to avoid that pain."
>
> —Julia Samuel, in *Grief Works: Stories of Life, Death, and Surviving*

My Four Counselors

Why did I have four grief counselors? If they were that good, wouldn't one do? Here's why:

1. **Rick Hobbs** was the counselor Hospice provided for a limited number of sessions. He lit a candle for Robert during our first meeting. He listened to my grief with great compassion and gentleness and gave me

hope. He told me he knew the light I had in me and I would find it again.

2. **Joe Hanson**, grief coach, now deceased, was a friend of a friend and in the right place at the right time. His daylong workshop, "The Power of Acceptance," catapulted me into a new understanding of my grief journey. Most meaningful was how I changed my story from "I lost the love of my life, and my life is and will be empty without him," to "I found the love of my life and learned how to experience love fully, and I take this with me on my path."

3. **Connie Kellogg** was the wise grief counselor provided by my HMO, Kaiser Permanente. She put me on Prozac temporarily for situational depression when I literally could not stop bawling. Her wise words, including "If you have a vibrator, it will work," (see Chapter 4, **Solo Sex**) helped me to rediscover my sexuality solo.

4. **Bill Roby** was my Kaiser therapist on an as-needed basis after Connie Kellogg retired. His wisdom, encouragement, and ability to articulate where I was on my grief journey and what strategies might work for me going forward meant the world to me during times I felt hopeless. He helped me prepare for special, grief-laden days like Robert's birthday and our wedding anniversary. Later, when I was vacillating, he encouraged me to try dating.

Do you need four grief counselors? Probably not, but in my opinion, you do need at least one. The grief journey is new to you, but it is the day job of these wonderful people. They will listen nonjudgmentally and share their understanding of where you are and what you might do to get to the next stage. They can offer coping strategies that have helped other people. They can suggest pharmaceutical help to blunt the searing pain.

Stages of Grief?

"Over the years, my grieving clients have come to see me for two reasons above all. First, given our death-phobic society, they felt like they had no other safe place to share the true feelings about their loss. Second, they were worried that they were going crazy. That concern was largely the by-product of theories like the stages of grief, which attempt to take a phenomenon that is natural, wholly unique, and unpredictable and make it into something diagnosable, like tonsillitis...Hard as it is to conceive now, there was a time when humans lived without the benefit of mental health professionals to pronounce whether they were grieving correctly."

—Patrick O'Malley, PhD, in *Getting Grief Right: Finding Your Story of Love in The Sorrow of Loss*

Yes, counselors and therapists can have an immense, positive effect—that's the point of this chapter. But be careful to choose one who understands that getting through grief isn't a lockstep process. You may go through the famous five "stages of grief"—the Kübler-Ross model: denial, anger, bargaining, depression, and acceptance—or you may experience grief differently. Elizabeth Kübler-Ross herself regretted using the word "stages" and wished she had used "aspects of grief" instead. Even if your process resembles these stages, it won't be a linear progression. You won't wake up one morning and say, "Okay, 'denial' is finished. On to 'anger.' " You'll likely cycle or spiral or bounce in and out of these and other emotions. It's all normal.

You may see your own process as four stages or six or ten, and you may swirl in and out of any of them. You won't progress neatly from one to another. Or you may feel (as I did) an intermingling hodgepodge of emotions that change without warning and can't be defined as "stages" at all.

A therapist who insists that there is one way the process works in predictable stages may make you feel that you're doing grief wrong. You're not.

What about Those Sexual Feelings?

I hope you'll feel comfortable talking to your counselor about your sexual feelings. Sex is part of wellness and part of being human. Even if sex isn't consciously on your mind and you can't imagine feeling whole enough for sex, your body will start to signal urges and needs, and eventually you'll crave release and the peace that brings, if only temporarily.

Don't avoid talking about these feelings with your counselor. At the least, you'll get reassurance that you're normal and that you're not betraying your deceased partner by having these urges and desires.

I was startled by this griever's story because her path and her feelings were so similar to mine:

A Griever Shares

I suffered an immeasurable loss when my husband, life partner, and soulmate of forty-two years died. In the early days, weeks, and months of my grieving, sex was the last thing on my mind. I was numb and sad, with bouts of impassioned praying, crying, and sobbing. I was on medications for migraine, depression, anxiety, and sleeplessness. I desperately missed his physical presence and his embrace as we lay in bed. I got a big body pillow to cuddle up to and, in the cold months, fell asleep with an herbal warming pad against me to simulate his warmth.

About six months after his passing, sexual feelings and longings began to return. I told my therapist that I was having some sexual feelings and was feeling ambivalent and confused. I guess I was looking for validation. She said that was all normal, and even suggested that I might want to get a vibrator—which I did. She also said it was perfectly normal—even healthy—to fantasize.

The first time I used the vibrator to make love to myself—imagining I was with him—I burst into tears afterward and just sobbed and sobbed. It felt so empty and unfulfilling. I missed him so much. My loneliness and grief were amplified. Then I went through a phase of pleasuring myself using my vibrator frequently. I imagined that I was with him and that we were making love as we used to when we were younger.

How Sex Coaching Can Help You with Grief

A perspective from Patti Britton, PhD, cofounder of SexCoachU.com, author of **Chasing Sex: Wanting Love, Finding Myself**

Working with a sex coach can help you address the natural evolution of your journey toward sexual wellness and wholeness. A sex coach helps you deal with your emotions, such as feelings of sadness, betrayal at being left behind, fear of the future, and worries about being alone the rest of your life without sex or touch. You'll learn to fill the empty space that your partner occupied with new, meaningful experiences and find joy from life itself, not just sexual pleasures or a new lover. A sex coach can help you heal the wounds that are now wide open and move forward from loss, grief, and the ultimate hardship of finding a new way to be as a sexual person.

Usually clients come to us when they've already done some of their critical healing work to become ready to face dating or become sexual again, alone or with a partner. Part of the focus might be to give yourself permission to engage in regular masturbation for pleasure and self-connection. By opening up the sexual channels, you may begin to feel pleasure, aliveness, and sexiness that might have been buried in the dung heap of your grief.

Focusing on small, self-care steps—physical, emotional, and social—can help you feel attractive to prospective new lovers, whether or not you take action in that direction. This focus can help to soothe the aching wounds of loneliness, awkwardness, and cluelessness about how to begin again in the world of dating and sexually connecting with new partners. We'll design action steps to help you overcome or resolve what is stopping you from what I call "sexual self-realization," which is about becoming fully who you can be as a sexual being.

Lessons from My Grief Counselors

I shared some excerpts from my Grief Journal in Chapter 15, **Journaling Your Journey.** I also took notes in that journal about what I learned from my grief counselors. I'm glad that I took those notes, and I recommend it to you. Counseling sessions can be so emotional and our grief brains so compromised, that without a written record, we may lose some of the best advice our counselors share.

Here are a few lessons I found particularly helpful:

- We don't get *over* grieving—we get *through* it.

- When the crying comes, give into it and don't try to stop it or numb yourself with a mindless activity. Let yourself experience your grief fully as it manifests itself now.

- For your birthday and other special days that make you miss your beloved most, create two new rituals—one that honors and affirms your connection to your beloved and another that is completely new and involves or helps other people.

- You don't get over grief, you get around it and around and around. Each time you circle around, it's a little easier, a little less intense.

- Be where you are when you're there. Let yourself experience your grief when it hits. At the same time, know that it's okay to seek out distraction when feeling exhausted from the grief itself. Grief is as much physical as it is mental and emotional.

- Dive into your grief and feel your way through it. The more energy you put into it, the faster it will move. Numbing yourself prolongs the process.

- Create an ongoing ritual or ceremony for your beloved that you will celebrate either on your own or with loved ones.

What If You Can't Afford Counseling?

If counseling doesn't seem within your budget, know that many licensed counselors and therapists see clients on a sliding scale and have limited openings for pro bono clients. Ask. Here are additional resources that can provide free or low-cost counseling and support groups:

- Your medical provider/health insurance

- Hospice

- Family services

- Pastoral counseling from your religious faith

- Support organization for your partner's medical condition, e.g. cancer center

- Mental health services

- Training programs for therapists through graduate schools and teaching hospitals

- Your job's Employee Assistance Program

- Online support groups

- Google "free or low-cost grief counseling near me."

"Will we open up and trust again? Will we let ourselves love again? And yes, openness is a choice. Everything in us wants to heal our loss and at the same time wants to be left alone with our grief, hoping that the pain may keep us connected to our loved one. We can stay closed down, or we can open up and share our struggle with someone who is qualified to walk with us on our journey...On our own, we will continue to veer off course, wearing down our inner resources...Only our yearning to be whole and healed can move beyond excuses/reasons into the office of a caring professional for realignment."

—Loretta McCarthy in *ABCs Of Grief: Reclaiming Life After Loss*

Your Takeaway

If you're not already seeing a grief counselor or
other professional, look into your local resources.
Ask a friend to help you locate resources if the
process seems too much to cope with right now.

CHAPTER 17

What's Next?

"The reality is that you will grieve forever. You will not 'get over' the loss of a loved one; you will learn to live with it. You will heal and you will rebuild yourself around the loss you have suffered. You will be whole again, but you will never be the same. Nor should you be the same nor would you want to."

—Elizabeth Kübler-Ross and David Kessler in
On Grief and Grieving

I n 2010, two years after Robert's death, I wrote this in *Naked at Our Age: Talking Out Loud about Senior Sex*:

"Although I couldn't imagine this at first, I'll have a lover again, and it will be good. I won't try to replace the love I shared with Robert— impossible—but there's a resiliency, a joy bubbling up that makes me feel vibrant and alive. Nurturing my sexual and loving self is a part of being fully alive that I will embrace, when it's time."

I had no idea when that time would come. I reflect on this now because I was starting to emerge from the hopelessness of grief into the next level, when hope was possible, when I could see that I had a future. We don't get over grief—but we do get through it. Somehow, we rise to the top and find ourselves again. When it's time—and no one can impose on you what the "right" time is—we may feel ready to let in someone new.

Grief While Poly

A perspective from Liz Powell, PsyD, psychologist, speaker, and author of **Building Open Relationships**

I was thirty-four years old when Elliot, my relatively new partner, died suddenly of a heart attack. For months afterward, I felt like I would fall apart if anyone touched me. Luckily, I had several great lovers who held space for me while I cried about the partner I had lost. Losing a partner while polyamorous is easier because of all the love and support you have available.

It's also challenging, because you don't want to overwhelm them with your grief, and you suddenly realize how many more intimate people you could lose. I find myself struggling with worries I never had before, wondering if something terrible happened when I don't hear back quickly from someone.

Overall, I think the death has helped me learn how to be more present in my relationships and how to ask for things from my partners more bravely.

My uncle, the celebrated psychotherapist Larry LeShan, went into the most profound grief when he lost his wife—child psychologist and author Eda LeShan—in 2002. They had been together for fifty-eight years. Knowing how deeply bereaved he was, I was surprised when he told me that he was in a new relationship with a woman whom he had known for years. "She brings color into my life," he told me. He still loved and missed Eda every moment. "Grief is a knife that never stops cutting," he said, "But over time, it cuts less often and less deeply." You, too, will be able to find color again.

If you're grieving deeply now, I don't want to offend you with the bright, chipper assurance that you will be all right—but I do believe that you will. Take your time. Let grief be your day job if that's how it feels to you. Confide in your friends. Make new friends. Send away anyone who tries to decide for you when your grief should end. It doesn't end, but it does soften.

When Sex Is Joyful Again

Grievers have written me with great surprise when sex with a new partner brought joy again. Sometimes it even brought love! Your new sexual partner is a gift, whether it lasts or not. We learn a lot about ourselves and our capacity for giving as well as receiving from our new relationships.

Let's end this book with experiences and reflections from grievers who have come out the other side and are, to their amazement, finding sexual exhilaration—even love—again:

Many Grievers Share

"Five weeks after my wife died, I had partnered sex with a marvelous widow of my age, seventy-three. This followed three years of my wife's ever-increasing decline and more than two years of no partnered sexual activity of any kind. I was grieving, but also immensely hungry for sexual arousal and touch beyond my regular self-pleasuring. That first sex means even more to me now, because that woman and I continue in a lively, joyous, and mutually supportive relationship—sexual and oh-so-much more—two years later."

*

"[I made] a few attempts at dating and sex after my husband died, and then I met the man I'm still with, a widower. We clicked. Eight years later, we still see each other a few times a week. We enjoy traveling together or just staying home, and without fail, we enjoy sex. Our bodies may be in their sixties, but our minds are young. Some positions need adjustments to allow for bad knees, but we don't mind. We never forget about our spouses, but they're not coming back. We're not disrespecting them. We mention them almost every time we're together."

*

"My darling was a sexy man. He gave my first orgasm and a new awareness and freedom of sex. He said, 'Sex is the cure-all!' This becomes my mantra when the old body's mind takes over and holds me back. I'm seventy-five and am now in a relationship with a man five years younger. My darling would have wanted me to be sexual with a new man. I feel him giving me permission for pleasure. Everyone grieves differently, and perhaps sex with a new man has been a gift, a surprise."

"More than six months have passed, and sex has gotten better and better. I need to start very gently and gradually go deeper as she relaxes. I love this 'slow sex.' Being aroused is a pleasure in itself, so I'm never in a hurry to reach orgasm. Orgasms are much better anyway when there is a slow buildup. Sex as a widower with my sexagenarian 'merry widow' is truly the best I've ever had."

*

"Sex felt so right for both of us, and it was more than I ever expected. We took it slow just to explore each other's bodies with touching. His wife had been sick for a long time, and he hadn't had sex in three years. I knew I needed patience for him to get and keep an erection. Patience has paid off in spades. We continue to explore each other inside and out. I am thankful that I kept my heart open and found a man whom I adore. No, sex isn't like when we were in our younger years, but I honestly think it is better in so many ways."

*

"Five years later, we are still together. Sex at this stage has been different. I have been more verbal and open in discussing my needs, and that is empowering. Achieving orgasm takes much longer. I still feel self-conscious getting naked with someone who never knew my young, lithe body. Yes, there can be sex after grief and loss. It will certainly be different, but it opens new opportunities for experimenting."

*

"I was widowed five years ago after forty-four years of a good marriage. After his death, my sexual needs continued. I masturbated and bought a vibrator. Six months ago, I started dating a widower. I was nervous our first time, but I responded to his kind, gentle patience. He told me later that he was very nervous too, which had never entered my mind. It shocked both of us how well we clicked sexually. He had been married fifty-two years and had been with no one else. Our love making now is amazing. We are in bed for hours. We've accepted each other's seventy-year-old bodies. He has ED, but we've overcome that with masturbation, oral sex, and toys. There is a heightened enjoyment and no rushing when we're together in bed. We talk, laugh, cuddle, and live for the moment, realizing it could all end at any time at our age. We're both so glad we took the risk to reach out and live life again."

*

"I wish someone could have communicated how much it hurts deep down to lose the love of one's life, but also that life goes on, and that one may be so fortunate as to find another person who fills that special role. I feel exceptionally lucky that this has happened to me, and I wish it for others who resume sex after grief as well."

"After my husband of forty-two years died two years ago, my life has been growth in many ways. His sudden death was overwhelming at first. I gave myself a year to work on myself with counseling, reflection, widow groups, journaling, and moving on as best I could. After the year, at sixty-seven, I put myself out there by joining Match.com. I really missed the intimacy, so I was open, cautiously, to the possibility that maybe there was someone out there for me. Then I got a message on Match from a man whose words and profile piqued my interest. He was a great communicator, and we seemed to have much in common. We have now been dating almost eleven months and I can't imagine my life without him. He is also a widower. His wife's death was only five months before we met, and this concerned me, but I kept my heart open. He told me later that I had him at hello."

*

"About fifteen months after my husband's passing, my friendship with one of my husband's oldest and dearest friends grew into an intimate one. He and I both embraced the idea of mutual exploration with no goal in mind. While our new sexual relationship is different than the one I had with my husband, I found that as part of the grieving process it's okay to be playful, laugh, and have fun again. I can't help but think that my dear loved one is looking at us from the 'other side' with approval and joy. It's never too late to rediscover yourself and your sexuality."

*

"I dated a man twenty years younger. When I orgasmed, he kept going! Once he decided to make me "come my age." I was forty-nine. I asked how he could count my orgasms when I could not tell when one ended and the next began. He explained that he was a trained mathematician."

Your Takeaway

What parts of this book were most valuable to you?
What did you learn that you can bring into your
life right now? What do you want to put into action
later? Make some notes now, whether you feel ready
to act on these ideas now or just think about them
until you're ready.

If this book was valuable to you, I'd love to hear
from you at joan@joanprice.com. Let me know
whether it's okay to share your comments—I won't
use your name or other identifying details—or
whether you'd like them to stay private between the
two of us.

CHAPTER 18

Better Sex

Y ou didn't think this could happen, but it does: You're dating someone new who attracts you, puts you at ease, makes you feel desirable. Lust chemicals flood your brain. You invite sex, maybe enthusiastically, maybe with reservations. It may feel awkward at first, but as you get to know each other's bodies, sex becomes hot and satisfying. You love being sexual again. You just wish your partner knew how to read your mind and know what you want, when, and how.

Mind reading: it doesn't work. Never did, never will. What *does* work? Talking out loud.

Good Sex Through Communication

A Griever Shares

"When I started dating, I told myself that if I was too uncomfortable to speak candidly about sex to a partner, we lacked the emotional intimacy to be having sex. I opened the conversation, and he welcomed it. We talked about physical and emotional needs and what actions in and out of the bedroom sparked our desire. We agreed on goals for frequency of sexual activity. We revisit the conversation as needs, desires, and physical abilities change. We've learned that spontaneity is overrated and scheduled sex dates are fun! Over ten years, our physical relationship has changed, and communication has been the key to a satisfying sex life."

Few of us learned how to talk to a partner about what we do and don't want sexually, especially in a loving and effective way. I've offered tips and scripts for talking about sex throughout this book and more in *Naked at Our Age: Talking Out Loud About Senior Sex*. Whether or not you communicated easily with your past partner, it's vital to practice doing that now.

Plus talking about sex can be erotic! "How would you like to be pleasured today?" is a sexy opening to a sexual encounter. That's what my partner and I say, and it's as arousing to express those words as to hear them!

When First Bloom Fades

Over time, the newness wears off. Even though you may feel more intimate with this new person, the raring-to-go, genitals-blazing feeling recedes. Your desire frequency or the kind of sex you want may be out of sync with your partner's. Orgasms are less dependable.

A Griever Shares

"What a delightful surprise to experience love again after grief and loss. Even more surprising, sexual intimacy at this stage of life was as exciting as in my younger years. It was great—until it wasn't. After the initial rush and thrill of new romance quieted, I still had a wonderful man I loved and was attracted to. I just didn't have the frequency of desire that matched his."

When Desire Happens Less Frequently

One of the most important concepts in sexuality is the difference between *spontaneous* and *responsive* desire. When you're new to each other, the desire for sex happens quickly, easily, spontaneously. Those lusty brain chemicals at work! But after being together for a time, you may feel more bonded, maybe in love, yet *spontaneous* desire isn't the driving force it once was.

That's a reason to learn about *responsive* desire: desire that arises *in response to* pleasure and physiological arousal. After we start feeling pleasure, our bodies start getting aroused, and *then* the desire *follows*.

A sign that this is your desire pattern is if you enjoy sex after you get started, but you don't particularly feel driven or desirous ahead of time. You love it once you get going, but you don't feel those urges *until* you start receiving pleasure. Then your body responds, your brain fires, and you're into it with relish. You may find yourself saying afterward, "Why don't we do this more often?"

Feeling spontaneous desire is *not* a requirement for great sex. Don't put off sex waiting for spontaneous desire—you'll just enjoy sexual pleasure much less often. Instead, plan your sexual encounters frequently, and leave time for slowly growing pleasure and arousal.

Learn more about responsive desire and women's arousal in Dr. Emily Nagoski's *Come As You Are: The Surprising New Science That Will Transform Your Sex Life*. Highly recommended!

What Does Good Sex Mean Now?

A Griever Shares

"As septuagenarians, our bodies don't respond like they did in our youth. Instead, we are unselfish lovers, concentrating most on pleasing each other. Our intimacy does not always lead to orgasm, but our sustained and gentle touching leads to unparalleled satisfaction. We are aware of life's fragility, and we treasure the true love we've found."

The secret to good sex is expanding your notion of what good sex is. The broader your definition, the better sex you'll have! This is crucial for older people, but also important for all ages. I described some options in "Expanding Sex Without Penetration" in Chapter 9, and you can be inventive about others. Concentrate on the pleasure you can give and receive, letting go of old notions about how sex is "supposed" to happen.

A Griever Shares

"I am a seventy-two-year-old man who lost my wife of forty-three years to cancer. I am impotent from prostate cancer surgery. My women friends encouraged me to start dating. 'What woman would want an impotent guy?' I asked them. They regaled me with tales of their many vagina problems, apparently not uncommon among seventy-something women. They said they want 'other things' sexually, not intercourse. Some older women still enjoy and crave penetrative sex, but, for many, impotence is not a bug—it's a feature! Don't be afraid to talk about it. Be open and respectful, and mature women will respond with kindness and empathy."

Exploring What Worked and What Didn't

Melanie Davis, PhD, AASECT-CSC, CSE; New Jersey Center for Sexual Wellness

If you had a great romantic or sexual connection with your past partner, you may be afraid to date now because you assume no one could compare. If your past relationship lacked something sexually, you may fear repeating that pattern.

If you've lost an amazing sexual partner, take heart that while you can't replicate the exact ways you two interacted, you know what worked well and can look for those qualities in a new relationship. For example:

- You spoke freely about your needs and interests.

- You were equally excited about each other's physical responses.

- You had similar ideas about shared pleasure, play, and communication.

If your relationship wasn't sexually satisfying, why not?

- Did your partner's pleasure take precedence over yours?
- Were your interests out of sync?
- Did you expect but not achieve sexual fireworks with your partner?
- Did you expect your partner to know how to turn you on without guidance, leading to disappointment?

As you get sexual with new partners, direct communication about sex is crucial. Learn to talk about the sexual activities you each enjoy or want to explore. Avoid performance pressure by focusing on sensual pleasures without goals. You may eventually see fireworks, but, even if you don't, you'll have plenty of fun experiences. If it goes well, you'll be on your way to the emotional and physical fulfillment you deserve.

CHAPTER 19

Two Loves

Embracing new love does not mean losing your heart connection with your deceased beloved. You can love both simultaneously. Every relationship is different, and if you bond with someone new, what happens between you reflects the two of you: your individual personalities, tempered by your histories, including your past experiences of love.

Cherish your memories along with your newfound happiness. By falling in love again—or wanting to—you're not falling out of love with the person who brought so much meaning into your life. Your heart can expand to love both. A new lover who's right for you will understand and welcome that.

Several Grievers Share

"My beloved wife died seven years ago, and our thirty-year relationship ended. Or did it? Her physical presence is gone. But her spirit and intellect permeate our home. She speaks to me every day. Her books, rose bushes, red geraniums, and favorite coffee mug comfort me. To my surprise, I met a widow who was very much like my wife: brainy, sexy, and saucy. She missed her beloved husband as deeply as I missed my wife, and this drew us together. From our first date on, we spoke about them openly and easily. Our feelings moved beyond the excitement of new relationship energy, and we tiptoed into love. That I also remain in love with my deceased wife doesn't bother my new heartthrob. She knows I celebrate her continued love for her deceased husband. Now we octogenarians are each blessed with two loves."

*

"My first husband was a longtime AIDS survivor. I am now remarried to another widower whose first husband also died of a terminal illness. We didn't rush into marriage, but our experience of the fragility of life led us to question, 'What are we waiting for?' Our deceased husbands are very much part of our lives. Their photos, artwork, and curios are displayed in our home. They are part of who we are now. Each of us occasionally experiences what we call 'landmines of grief.' But with the tears come understanding and compassion. We share a depth of sexual intimacy, spontaneity, and freedom. Communication is key, including frankly sharing experiences with our late husbands."

*

"My wife died after fifty years together. I had the good fortune to meet a lovely woman of my age, also widowed after a long and loving marriage. It took a long time to relearn courtship activities—like holding hands! But from the start we were comfortable talking about our beloved lost spouses. It was a surprise to learn that we could find new love and not feel that we were betraying our lost loves, or even forgetting them for a moment. We tell each other that we will never stop loving our spouses—and that they must have set us up!"

> "Polyamory gave me the framework to love others while still honoring the person I lost. It became fluid and easy to give my loss partner her place without losing her—she is my base with other partners added on. It works so well this way."

LAT (Living Apart Together)

You lived a life with your partner. Then you learned to live alone. It was hard at first, but as time passed, you discovered that you like your solitude and independence. Now you're in love again. Does committing to a new relationship mean you're expected to marry or move in together? Which of the special photos, gifts, or memory-filled objects can you display in a home you share with a new lover? You worry that creating a household with your new person will push your connection to your deceased partner into the background.

Here's another option: Living Apart Together (LAT). You can be a committed couple and choose to live separately, spending time together—including overnights—when you wish. LAT is increasingly popular with widowed people with their own homes, habits, and finances. You can love another person and still choose to "Live Close By, Visit Often," as K.T. Oslin sings.

In Chapter 3, I wrote about being two years into a new relationship in "And When It Works…" We just celebrated our seventh anniversary—in a LAT arrangement. Because we don't live together, our relationship doesn't get stale or predictable. When it's been a while, we're really glad to see each other. And then we're really glad to be on our own again, in the houses filled with reminders of our deceased spouses. LAT isn't for everyone, but every time I describe this relationship style to an audience, several people say, "I didn't know that was a thing! Sign me up!"

Several Grievers Share

"We've been in a loving, monogamous relationship—happily unmarried—for ten years now. We own homes nearby and get together several times a week. After dating for a year, we shared a vacation condo for two months, our first experience living together. We had a good time, but constant togetherness highlighted some fundamental differences. We enjoyed returning to our own separate houses. We realized that marriage would complicate more than enhance our relationship. We value both our independence and commitment to each other. This way, we have the best of both."

*

"Despite my women friends encouraging me to go on dating sites, I couldn't bring myself to do it. One of these friends was my massage therapist, whom I've known for nine years. We became friends, then closer than friends. She did the professional thing and fired me as a client—then rehired me as her boyfriend! We have no interest in getting married or living together, but we love one another the best that we can."

*

"I am a widower in a relationship with a widow. We live apart together. My home is replete with memorabilia of my deceased wife. My partner's is full of reminders of her beloved husband. Neither of us finds these loving memories threatening to our happiness together. We often share tales about what made our former spouses so special to us. We recognize that we are not in competition with those who preceded us."

And While We Wait...

"Lately, I've had a surprise visitor: my late husband, Jerry. I am feeling his love for me all over again, twenty-eight years after his death. I feel a closeness with him again and a deep appreciation for how much he loved me. This gives me hope of finding someone else with similar qualities who wants to share passion, excitement, and sexual pleasure with me."

—Lynn Brown Rosenberg, author of *My Sexual Awakening at 70: And What Led Me Here*

"My wife was amazing. Absolutely amazing. But the truth is she is not the only amazing woman to be born. As I hope to fall in love again one day, I don't compare new love interests to her. That would be a disservice to them. To me. And to her. She was one in seven billion. Just as I am. Just as you are. There will never be another Michelle. Just as there will never be another John. Or another "John & Michelle." When looking for love again, I'm not looking for another Michelle. I'm looking to find another human, whom I adore."

—John Polo, *The Stupid Sh*t People Say to Grievers*

CHAPTER 20

When Life
Throws Curveballs

I invited grievers from the 2019 edition of *Sex After Grief* to tell me where they are now, what has happened since they first wrote. I also invited new grievers to send their stories of inviting sex into their lives. Many stories were filled with hope and new connections. Some were not. Life sends us curveballs, and this book would be less than truthful if I omitted those.

If you're experiencing setbacks like these or a different kind, take comfort in knowing that you're not alone. Please seek counseling to help you through this tough time. And treasure the good memories.

When Joy Is Short-Lived

A Griever Shares

"It has been eight years since my husband died
and one year since my boyfriend passed away.
My husband sucked the life out of me. My
boyfriend gave it back. We first hooked up in the
'70s and married others. After my husband died,
he reentered my life—my sexual awakening! I
nicknamed him 'BLE': Best Lover Ever. When I
masturbate, I still conjure him up."

When Robert died after only seven years together,
a close male friend told me, "I don't think I could
risk falling in love again and losing my lover like
you did." He had witnessed my tears and listened
to my stories. He didn't think love was worth
that heartache.

"It was worth it to love and be loved by Robert,
however temporary it turned out to be," I told
him. "I'd do it all over again, even knowing how
it would end." Sometimes the joy is short-lived,

but it's all we get to have. The love is worth
the suffering.

A Griever Shares

"My husband died after suffering with
Alzheimer's for fifteen years. I'd been working
and caring for him. I started dating and at
seventy-five, I married a wonderful guy. I felt like
a new person. Sex was so much fun. Then poof:
a prostate cancer diagnosis. Radiation therapy
followed while we held our breath and prayed.
He survived! But cancer treatment swept away
his libido and our sex life. Two years passed
with daily kisses but no sex. Our relationship
suffered. Could I stay without feeling desired?
We found two wonderful counselors: a marriage
counselor and a sex therapist, both older women
with life experience in addition to training. They
are saving our marriage. I am hopeful about our
future and look forward to having fun with sex
again. It will be different from what I've been
used to, but that is okay. We now have help."

Grief Bursts

A Griever Shares

"My wife adored donkeys. We owned a cabin on rural property an hour's drive from our home. We drove there frequently for the quietude and beauty. En route was a small farm with two donkeys. She always watched for them and exclaimed, 'There they are!' The donkeys became a special joy we anticipated. I sold our rural property soon after my wife died. My grief diminished from tears and heartache to a dull pain as the years passed. I happened to travel that road again recently. The two donkeys were peacefully grazing, as if nothing had changed. 'There they are!' I exclaimed. I began weeping so uncontrollably that I had to pull over to gather myself. When we've lost our beloved, grief always lies just below the surface. It can jolt us at wholly unexpected moments."

We can be doing fine, adjusting to our "new normal," even loving again. Then pow! Something reminds us of a special time with our beloved, and we're gut-punched. This used to happen to me frequently. Now it's rare, but still powerful. I find it works best if I let myself fully experience the burst and honor it as a sign that our love is still within me.

I Can't Date Yet

A Griever Shares

"My husband was diagnosed with cancer five months after our first date. He died five years later. I was heartbroken. Months after his death, I craved a man's touch. I didn't feel ready to be with another man, so I decided to wait until the twelve-month mark. At that point, though, my grief felt worse! The fog of Year One lifted, and Year Two slammed me with the permanence of his death. Dating was the last thing on my mind. I'm now seven years out and still haven't dated. It's not that I don't want to. Life has thrown me some large curveballs and dating is low priority. However, the time and challenges have taught me a lot about myself. I now have a clearer vision of what I want in a partner, and for my future."

Grief has no predetermined or predictable timeline, nor does readiness to get sexual with a new partner. I've discussed this throughout this book. Give yourself permission to take as long as it takes. Realize that the waiting time is also a time of growth and self-knowledge.

Guilt

A Griever Shares

"There are worse kinds of bereavement than death. I live in a state of renewed bereavement every day because my ninety-year-old wife lives permanently in a care home suffering from vascular dementia. I wake up each morning suffering her loss. I go to bed each night to find that there's no warm bottom to spoon. I suffer guilt as I go on dating sites looking for a new sex partner. It's a battle between hormones and my marriage vows, and I'm afraid that hormones are going to win. I'm beating myself up because I feel I'm betraying my wife of seventy years, whom I still love. The feeling of shame does not bode well for any relationship."

Many grievers express guilt about seeking sex with a new person. They feel they're betraying their partner who is either deceased or no longer capable of an intimate relationship. Ask yourself: If the situation was reversed, what would you want for your beloved? Never to love or be happy again? To stay stuck in mourning, alone forever? Of course not.

Now imagine what your partner would tell *you*. If there was real love, I think you'd hear, "Find pleasure and happiness again. Find love again. Don't shut down."

If you are fortunate enough to have your partner with you now, give this great gift to each other.

Say, "If I die before you, or we can no longer be a couple, I want you to find joy with someone else." I wish every couple would have this conversation.

Reflections

Ann Anderson Evans, author of **The Sweet Pain of Being Alive: A Memoir of Love and Death**

I'm fine. I sleep well, eat well, play pickleball and walk the dog, have friends, groups, interests, am inspired by Nature, and am watching the basketball playoffs.

I only maintain this equilibrium if I stay away from sex and romance. My husband Terry, who feels like my only husband (the two others didn't hold a candle), killed himself in May 2020, going on five years ago.

During the first four years, I was a widow— it was life without Terry as opposed to life with Terry. Then along came a man who courted me for a while and made love to me. I was relieved that I could have sex again, but his presence struck deep into my sense of loss, of failure, of confusion. I cut it off.

To get healthier, I wanted other men's voices to dilute Terry in my head. So I joined a few dating sites and accomplished that goal. But I still have difficulty going deeper than laughter and chatter.

My daily assignment is to do everything for the first time. The great arches of religion, family, work, citizenship, relationship, and so on are built on a million first times. I don't know what I'm building right now, but I'm, as I said, fine.

CHAPTER 21

Moving Forward

Moving on from grief doesn't mean letting go of your beloved's place in your heart. Your heart is big enough to hold your deceased dear one, an ever-expanding sense of your own self, and space for another, should you decide to let someone in.

Here are some helpful expert tips to guide you, followed by stories from grievers about how they found love again—often with surprising realizations!

New Beginnings: Who Are You, Who Do You Want to Be?

Dr. Linda Kirkman, Australia-based sexologist, www.lindakirkman.org

Take the time to reflect on your sexual expression and relationships to date. Ask yourself:

- What has worked well for me, felt right?

- What would I like to express differently, including my sexuality and gender identity?

- What have I not explored that I'd like to explore, such as fantasies and unmet desires?

If you feel ready for a new relationship or relationships, consider who you are now, what awesomeness you bring to a new relationship, and what you need. You may want things that didn't fit with your last partner, so you didn't pursue them. Maybe now is the time to find someone who shares these interests, beliefs, and desires. If new beginnings feel daunting, find a therapist you feel safe with to explore what you might like to change.

Filling the Hole with Love

Charlie Glickman, PhD, somatic sexuality & relationship coach, www.makesexeasy.com

Many people describe grief as a hole in their heart, a feeling of deep loss. Talking about the person who died, focusing on what you loved about them, can kind of patch that hole with the love and help you move through the grief. If you find yourself focusing on how you miss them, bring it back to what you loved about them. It's not about wallowing in grief. It's about celebrating who they were in your life and how you felt about them.

Embrace Change

Carolyn Gower, grief coach and educator,
My Person Died Too *podcaster, www.*
carolyngowercoaching.com

My widowed clients often want a carbon copy of their late partner when they start dating again. Some seek qualities they found attractive in their partner when they first met, though that might have been ten, twenty, or thirty years ago. Spending a lot of time together in a romantic relationship moulded you into the unique people you became within that relationship. Realize that you were only those versions of yourselves *with each other*. Expecting someone else to slot right into their place leads to disappointment.

Both of you changed over your time together, and you've continued to change since your loss. Who are you now, on your own? I see many clients who experience post-traumatic growth and want completely different things in a partner post-loss. What are the attributes you want in a partner now?

Never Too Late for New Love

Several Grievers Share

"I'm sixty-three and a widow of seven years. I've dated some nice men, but with no spark of attraction, no stirring to connect intimately. I was content with my Magic Wand. Then I met Joey! When Joey kissed me. I felt warmth spreading within me that had been long dormant. My whole body buzzed. We've been nearly inseparable since we met. I can't imagine how I would have managed COVID quarantine without this relationship. Joey is actually Josephine, a beautiful, lively woman of my age. I've never been attracted to a woman before and never would have predicted this. Call me 'Surprised Widow!' "

*

"My wife of forty-eight years passed away after dealing with multiple sclerosis and nine years as a quadriplegic. It had been many years without sex. After months of mourning, I tried to mitigate loneliness by signing up for online dating, joining the Senior Center, and enrolling in classes. Serendipitously at a hospice function, I sat with a lady I had met in a class. Our conversation led to a date, then many others. When she first reached to hold my hand, I felt a rush of emotion, realizing how I missed physical contact. That touch ignited a desire for closeness that had been missing in my life. Our odyssey together progressed like we were teenagers again: butterflies when we saw one another, warm and frequent hugs, gentle kisses, then overnighters. Intimacy became an important part of our relationship as our deep love grew."

*

"I took the plunge and decided to seek competent help rather than muddle through my grief. I moved forward with the support of an extraordinary professional surrogate partner. She mended and mentored my progress back into life. I learned that progress does not mean moving on from what you had, but moving forward with what you have now. I now have two loving polyamorous partners who enrich my life beyond my expectations. You do not leave your love behind—you build additions to it, while keeping that past love alive and vibrant."

*

"I was my wife's caregiver for ten years before she died. Six months later, I realized that I couldn't live alone. I craved human companionship. Sexual thoughts haunted my nights. Then I found her online. She lived half a continent away. Her emergence from grief mirrored mine. Within two weeks we were doing things on FaceTime that we hoped no internet snoop could see. Thirty-eight days after our first online meeting, I flew to her. She was petite, stylish, beautiful. She felt warm and cuddly under my arm. She folded herself into me. Sharing our first kiss, her tongue was sweet, warm, and soft, and it left me trembling. Our first sexual encounter was awkward and delicious. Someone wanted me as much as I wanted her! Two and a half years later, we're still lovers. We make long, languid love every day we're together. My advice? Carpe diem. You may not have another."

Looking Back—and Forward

For many months after Robert died, I started each morning writing in my memory journal, surrounded by his paintings, sipping coffee from the special mug he'd use for bringing me coffee in bed. As much as grief ripped my heart every day, all day, part of me feared moving on. If I lost the deep grief, would I also lose the memories? Would his beautiful face and body fade? Would I no longer remember his voice, his scent, his touch?

It's been sixteen years since Robert's death as I write this. I still see his face, his body in motion, but no longer in sharp focus. The handle broke off the special mug, and I can't use it for hot coffee anymore. But Robert's paintings and gifts are still on display in every room. Each time I dance at home, I reverently touch his note with "Dancing with you!" in his handwriting under a painted heart. My memories still fill me, even though they have softened.

At eighty-one, I'm living a full and joyful life personally, professionally, intellectually, and romantically. Robert still lives in me, and the love we shared gives color and dimension to everything else in my life. I feel him nodding in approval as I write this.

Thank you for sharing this journey with me.

About the Author

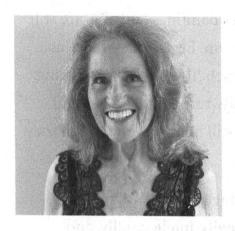

J oan Price, joanprice.com, calls herself an advocate for ageless sexuality. She is known by American and global media as the voice of senior sex. Her award-winning blog has offered senior sex news, views, and sex toy reviews since 2005. Age eighty-one at the time of this second edition, Joan continues to talk out loud about senior sex— partnered or solo.

Joan is an internationally known speaker and educator on older-age sexuality. She speaks to groups as varied as seniors, therapists, health professionals, sexuality conferences, sex toy shops, and college students. Some popular presentations are available as webinars from joanprice.com.

Joan Price has been writing the monthly "Ask Joan" sex and relationships advice column for SeniorPlanet.org since 2014. She is the collaborator, script writer, and narrator of *jessica drake's Guide to Wicked Sex: Senior Sex*, which won the Audiovisual Award 2020 from American Association of Sexuality Educators, Counselors and Therapists (AASECT).

Joan's other sexuality books include:

- *Naked at Our Age: Talking Out Loud About Senior Sex*, winner of Outstanding Self-Help Book 2012 from American Society of Journalists and Authors and 2012 Book Award from American Association of Sexuality Educators, Counselors, and Therapists

- *Better Than I Ever Expected: Straight Talk about Sex After Sixty*, Joan's spicy memoir about her love story with artist Robert Rice, celebrating the joys of older-age sexuality

- *The Ultimate Guide to Sex After 50: How to Maintain—or Regain!—a Spicy, Satisfying Sex Life*, Joan's most comprehensive senior sex book, addressing how to overcome the challenges of sex and changing relationships

- *Ageless Erotica*, a steamy senior sex anthology which Joan conceived and edited, featuring sexy characters over fifty, from writers over fifty

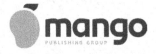

Mango Publishing, established in 2014, publishes an eclectic list of books by diverse authors—both new and established voices—on topics ranging from business, personal growth, women's empowerment, LGBTQ+ studies, health, and spirituality to history, popular culture, time management, decluttering, lifestyle, mental wellness, aging, and sustainable living. We were named 2019 *and* 2020's #1 fastest growing independent publisher by *Publishers Weekly*. Our success is driven by our main goal, which is to publish high-quality books that will entertain readers as well as make a positive difference in their lives.

Our readers are our most important resource; we value your input, suggestions, and ideas. We'd love to hear from you— after all, we are publishing books for you!

Please stay in touch with us and follow us at:

Facebook: Mango Publishing
Twitter: @MangoPublishing
Instagram: @MangoPublishing
LinkedIn: Mango Publishing
Pinterest: Mango Publishing

Newsletter: mangopublishinggroup.com/newsletter

Join us on Mango's journey to reinvent publishing, one book at a time.